AGEING and
LONG-TERM CARE

National
Policies
in the
Asia-Pacific

The **Asian Development Research Forum** (ADRF) is a development research management / policy research networking group focused on East, Southeast and South Asia, now managed by the Thailand Research Fund (TRF) with major support from the International Development Research Centre (IDRC), Canada. Since the ADRF's establishment in 1997, its focus has been to strengthen Policy Synthesis in three main areas; (1) Ageing Asian Populations; (2) Asian Economic and Financial Governance; and (3) Asian Conflict Management. Its working group manages each main area. In July 2002, the ADRF broadened this focus to include the areas of Policy Synthesis and Community Empowerment in Environmental Management. The ADRF is unique in that it provides an Asian, cross-national (regional) view and is forward-looking.

The **International Development Research Centre** (IDRC) is a public corporation created by the Parliament of Canada in 1970 to help developing countries use science and technology to find practical, long-term solutions to the social, economic, and environmental problems they face. Support is directed towards developing an indigenous research capacity to sustain policies and technologies developing countries need to build healthier, more equitable, and more prosperous societies. IDRC's catalogue of publications is available at <www.idrc.ca/booktique>.

The **Institute of Southeast Asian Studies (ISEAS),** Singapore, was established as an autonomous organization in 1968. It is a regional research centre for scholars and other specialists concerned with modern Southeast Asia, particularly the many-faceted problems of stability and security, economic development, and political and social change. The Institute's research programmes are the Regional Economic Studies (RES, that includes ASEAN and APEC), Regional Strategic and Political Studies (RSPS), and Regional Social and Cultural Studies (RSCS). ISEAS' catalogue of publications is available at <www.iseas.edu.sg/pub.html>.

AGEING and LONG-TERM CARE

National Policies in the Asia-Pacific

Edited by
David R. Phillips & Alfred C.M. Chan

Institute of Southeast Asian Studies
Singapore

International Development Research Centre
Canada

Published in cooperation with the
Asian Development Research Forum
and the
Thailand Research Fund
Thailand

Published jointly by the
Institute of Southeast Asian Studies
30 Heng Mui Keng Terrace, Pasir Panjang
Singapore 119614
<www.iseas.edu.sg/pub.html>
ISBN 981-230-173-9

and the
International Development Research Centre
PO Box 8500
Ottawa, ON K1G 3H9
Canada
<www.idrc.ca>
ISBN 1-55250-005-5

in cooperation with the
Asian Development Research Forum
<www.adrf.org>

© 2002 Thailand Research Fund
<www.trf.or.th>

ISEAS Library Cataloguing-in-Publication Data

Ageing and long-term care: national policies in the Asia-Pacific / edited by
David R. Phillips and Alfred C.M. Chan.
(Social Issues in Southeast Asia)
    1. Ageing—Government policy—Asia.
    2. Aged—Care—Asia.
    I. Phillips, David R. (David Rosser), 1953-
    II. Chan, Alfred C. M.
    III.   Series.
HQ1064 A9A261   2002   sls2002023106

ISBN 981-230-173-9 (soft cover)

Typeset by International Typesetters Pte. Ltd.
Printed and bound in Singapore by Bestprint Printing Co.

Contents

List of Figures

List of Tables

List of Contributors

Alfred Chan Cheung-ming
Asia–Pacific Institute of Ageing Studies and
Department of Politics and Sociology
Lingnan University
Hong Kong

Napaporn Chayovan
College of Population Studies
Chulalongkorn University
Bangkok
Thailand

Sung-Jae Choi
Department of Social Welfare
Seoul National University
Seoul
Korea

Sutthichai Jitapunkul
Faculty of Medicine
Chulalongkorn University
Bangkok
Thailand

Jiraporn Kespichayawattana
Faculty of Nursing
Chulalongkorn University
Bangkok
Thailand

Kalyani K. Mehta
Department of Social Work and Psychology
Faculty of Arts and Social Sciences
National University of Singapore
Singapore

Ong Fon Sim
Faculty of Business and Accountancy
University of Malaya
Kuala Lumpur
Malaysia

David R. Phillips
Asia–Pacific Institute of Ageing Studies and
Department of Politics and Sociology
Lingnan University
Hong Kong

Preface

This book is the result of a three-year collaboration under the Asian Development Research Forum's (ADRF) Ageing Research Network. It represents the collaborative efforts of researchers in gerontology in five countries in the Asia–Pacific region, the first stage of a continuing review of national policies on ageing and older persons in the region. The ADRF is a network of researchers based primarily in the Asia–Pacific region and Canada and was established under the auspices of Canada's International Development Research Centre (IDRC) in 1997. A number of meetings have been hosted since 1997 to focus on the various sub-groups' interests, held in Hong Kong, Seoul, Kuala Lumpur, Singapore, the Philippines and Thailand. From 2002 to 2005, the Thailand Research Fund (TRF) is managing the ADRF with major funding support from the IDRC. We wish to warmly acknowledge the IDRC's help and support in all these ventures for the ADRF and the TRF's continuing management of the Forum. The ADRF brings together researchers, policy-makers, research managers, government organizations and NGOs in the region, to focus on interconnected, interdisciplinary research areas of policy relevance to the region and its constituent member states. The forum's overall aim is "to increase the impact of development research in Asia through collaboration, policy innovation and balancing the social, economic and environmental imperatives". Three principal areas of interest have evolved: economic and financial governance, conflict resolution, and the socio-economic and political impacts of ageing. More details may be seen on the ADRF's website <www.adrf.org>.

As editors, we owe a great deal to the promptness of the contributors to this volume and to other members of the ADRF

Ageing Research Network, whose country studies will appear in future publications. In the wider context, we particularly wish to acknowledge the wisdom of Dr Randy Spence, then Regional Director of IDRC in its Singapore office, who founded the ADRF. The Forum's development has continued under the guidance of his successor, Dr Stephen McGurk. Many IDRC staff have been involved and we would like particularly to thank Tan Say-Yin and Martin Bazelwych of the IDRC Singapore Office who have given invaluable input to the administration of the ADRF. Elsewhere, Professor Chia Siow Yue, Director of the Institute of Southeast Asian Studies (ISEAS), deserves special mention for her support of the meeting of the ADRF in June 2001, when the plans for the book were finalized, and for her support for its publication by ISEAS in Singapore. The previous Chair of the ADRF, Professor Sieh Mei-ling of the University of Malaya and her successor as Chair, Dr Vicharn Panich, Special Adviser to the Thailand Research Fund (TRF), have been very supportive of the Forum as a whole and of the Ageing Research Network in particular. Many other people have contributed to the appearance of this volume, including our colleagues in the Asia–Pacific Institute of Ageing Studies, Lingnan University, especially Fanny Fung, Luk Kit-ling and Helen Lau.

In terms of content, this book was written by members of the ADRF's Ageing Research Network, which is coordinated from the Asia–Pacific Institute of Ageing Studies in Lingnan University, Hong Kong. It focuses on five case-study countries, which feature alphabetically in the contents: Hong Kong, Korea, Malaysia, Singapore and Thailand. These countries have a considerable range in population sizes (from Thailand's 63 million to Singapore's 4 million in 2001) and also in geographical area. Nevertheless, they share certain regional and cultural features, especially their philosophies of family support and the value of older persons in society. They are also all facing the similar phenomenon of demographic ageing (whereby populations age gradually, mainly from falling fertility rates and longer expectation of life). The ageing of populations poses challenges to governments, families and societies the world over. This is especially so in certain countries of the Asia–Pacific region, as

Asia has over half of the world's people aged 65 and above (Population Reference Bureau 2001). Many of these people live in countries in the Asia–Pacific area of the Asian region. The book therefore focuses on fundamental questions related to the development, or non-development, of coherent national policies on ageing and the long-term care for older persons. These questions and the major issues to be addressed in the book are outlined in Chapter 1.

As editors, we would also like to give a few notes on the terminology used in the book. First, we refer to the five case studies as "countries", although strictly speaking this applies to only four, as Hong Kong since July 1997 has been a Special Administrative Region (SAR) of the People's Republic of China. Singapore, too, is more generally referred to as a city–state, although it is an independent sovereign entity. Second, we generally refer to "older persons", "senior citizens" or "elderly people", which are today more accepted appropriate terms than "the elderly". We tend to use "the elderly " only when it refers to population segments such as cohorts aged (say) 65 and over, or to legislation or specific titled services in the countries in question.

David R. Phillips and Alfred Chan Cheung-ming
Asia–Pacific Institute of Ageing Studies (APIAS)
Lingnan University
Hong Kong
March 2002

Please visit the following web sites:
APIAS: <www.LN.edu.hk/apias>
Asian Development Research Forum: <www.adrf.org>
Thailand Research Fund: <www.trf.or.th>

1

National Policies on Ageing and Long-term Care in the Asia–Pacific Issues and Challenges

David R. Phillips & Alfred C. M. Chan

Introduction

The principal aim of this book is to provide a detailed review of the progress and prospects for the development of national policies on ageing and for older persons in selected countries of the Asia–Pacific region. Most countries of the region are ageing quite rapidly in demographic terms, although this is slower in some countries than in others. This demographic ageing of the populations is also occurring in quite dramatically changing social and economic contexts, and some cultural traditions are affecting the nature of policies for older persons.

The selection of countries represents a geographic and demographic spread across the region and, whilst representative, it cannot claim to be comprehensive. The book will not go in to great detail about the nature of and factors underlying demographic change in the region or in the case-study countries, Hong Kong, Korea, Malaysia, Singapore and Thailand. It will cover in general terms these factors, as they have important socio-economic consequences (lower fertility rates, smaller families, increasing life expectancy and the like). For a more comprehensive discussion of the underlying demographic dimensions in the Asia–Pacific region and elsewhere, readers may refer to Kinsella (2000), Kinsella and Velkoff (2001) and HelpAge International (2002).

Instead of focusing on demographic details, the case-study chapters address a number of key issues with regard to national policies on ageing and the provision of long-term care. The handling of these key issues is tailored to each case-study country as appropriate, rather than being treated in a mechanical manner, as the evolution of general policy regarding older persons, and long-term care in particular, is at different stages, and evolving from different contexts, in each country. Prior to outlining the key issues addressed, some basic definitions of national policies and long-term care may be presented.

First, we consider that "policy" may be taken to mean the development of a coherent conceptual framework linking different practices for the achievement of a goal or mission — in this case addressing "ageing" or older persons. Given this definition, the gradual development of such a policy framework has been evident in most of the case-study countries over the past two to three decades. However, practice in each country has not always matched policy, and services and support have therefore not always been consistent with national policies on ageing.

Secondly, long-term care must be considered, as it underpins the entire nature of provision for older persons, especially in later life. Traditionally, many authorities have regarded long-term care (LTC) as comprising mainly residential care services such as nursing homes, homes for the aged and hospital geriatric beds (Kahana 2000). This is a rather narrow view and has tended to focus attention on the more dependent members of the older population. It has tended to neglect the broader welfare and social support needs of currently active older persons, especially those living in the community, alone or with family members or in some other group settings. A broader view of LTC encompasses the range of support services that will help such people to live independently or with their families.

Given that "long-term care" has many different interpretations, we take a much broader definition of LTC as the starting position for consideration of policy and practice in this area. We take LTC to include "the full range of health, personal care and social services provided at home and in the community for a continuing period to adults who lack or have lost the capacity to care fully for themselves and remain independent" (Phillips 2000a, p. 1652). Indeed, the term can include services that are provided to reasonably fit and active older persons that enable them to remain living in the community, and who might otherwise lead lives that are less full and of lower quality, or even become institutionalized. Therefore, it is clear under this definition that certain community care and support systems, such as day care centres, home nursing and home helper services, can be included in the discussion (Hutten and Kerkstra 1996). There is also a very important aspect of evaluation of older persons' needs for LTC, bearing in mind that some older persons' who score similarly on many of the rating scales might in practice have different LTC needs because of their social and economic circumstances. Some might have extensive family or friendship support networks, or private resources to employ assistance. Other people may be more isolated and economically poorer, meaning that they will be far more reliant on local LTC support. In addition, it is crucial to be aware that older persons' needs (indeed, the needs of people in any age group) can change suddenly and sometimes dramatically. Therefore, part of the challenge of devising LTC policy and provision is to develop responsive, accessible and flexible provision. This is a major challenge in several of the case-study countries.

The regional context for national policies on ageing

These five case-study countries are members of the United Nations Economic and Social Commission for Asia and the Pacific (ESCAP), and as such their experience of developing national policies on ageing can be viewed in a regional context. The ESCAP region has taken a long-term view of the causes and consequences of ageing in a wide sphere of activities, and has placed this view in the context of regional development. Indeed, the region has been very active in considering and reviewing policies regarding ageing for some time, and has prepared the *Macau Plan of Action on Ageing for Asia and the Pacific* (*Macau POA*, ESCAP 1999). This provides a set of concise recommendations and specific guidelines, forming a framework within which individual countries can set their own goals and targets. The Plan of Action draws on the 1982 Vienna International Plan of Action on Ageing, the 1992 Proclamation on Ageing of the United Nations, and various other internationally agreed principles. The *Macau POA* has been reviewed and discussed extensively in regional consultation meetings in preparation for the Second World Assembly on Ageing held in Spain in April 2002. The *Macau POA* identified a number of wide areas of concern stemming from socio-economic and demographic changes that are affecting all countries. Phillips and Chan have conducted a review for ESCAP (ESCAP 2001*a*) of the critical issues in national policies and programmes on ageing in the region, as highlighted in the *Macau POA* and the *United Nations International Plan of Action on Ageing*, developed in anticipation of the UN International Year of Older Persons in 1999 (United Nations 1998). As planned, the progress of the implementation of the *Macau POA* has been monitored, and data were received and collated from the responses of 25 countries to a questionnaire prepared by the ESCAP secretariat. This interim review of progress provides an important snapshot on the region (ESCAP 2001*b*) and is being repeated in 2002.

The concerns of the *Macau POA* are underpinned by the dramatic demographic transformation resulting from the combined effects of mortality and fertility reduction and the dramatic increase in the proportion of older persons. By the end of the first quarter of this century, the proportion of the population aged 60 and over will reach 20–25 per cent or more in certain countries such as Japan, Australia, New Zealand and the Republic of Korea. In other countries, such as China, India and the Philippines, the concern is not so much with the proportion of older persons to the rest of the population, but with their absolute numbers, given the huge population bases of some ESCAP countries. It is also important to realize that this demographic transition is occurring within the context of numerous changes in national institutions and values, because of rapid social and economic development. Traditional institutions such as the family and community are undergoing concomitant changes, and they may no longer be able to fulfil their traditional support roles. The *Macau POA* addressed seven specific areas of concern relating to ageing and older persons in the Asia–Pacific region, all of which are relevant to the development of national policies on ageing and long-term care in the countries covered in this book:

1. The social position of older persons
2. Older persons and the family
3. Health and nutrition
4. Housing, transportation and the built environment
5. Older persons and the market
6. Income security, maintenance and employment
7. Social services and the community

The Second World Assembly on Ageing, Madrid 2002, produced the *Madrid International Plan of Action on Ageing 2002*. This grouped many international issues and areas of concern under three "priority directions": I Older persons and development; II Advancing health and well-being into old age; and III Ensuring enabling and supportive environments (United Nations 2002). These areas of concern relate closely to those identified in the *International Plan of Action on Ageing and United Nations Principles for Older Persons* developed in anticipation of the International Year of Older Persons (United Nations 1998), which were:

1. Health and nutrition
2. Protection of elderly consumers
3. Housing and environment
4. Family
5. Social welfare
6. Income security and employment
7. Education

From these reviews, Phillips and Chan (ESCAP 2001*a*) identified several key areas of concern in the development of national policies (long-term care itself being one of these key areas). First was the importance of social participation of older persons, including the stereotyping of older people in many parts of the region. Second, older persons have to be considered within the changing nature of traditional support systems and shifting intergenerational relationships. Third, a challenge is to develop appropriate environments especially the built environment, for older persons, and to provide access to services, which is crucial to successful ageing within the community "ageing in place", otherwise known as a policy discussed later in this chapter. Fourth, accommodation and long-term care form key issues of concern, and are closely linked to the fifth area, epidemiological transition, which emphasizes the importance of developing comprehensive primary health care and welfare services. Finally, a key issue underpinning all national policies is that of income security, maintenance and employment, the challenge of poverty in old age, and the feminization of poverty, as many more women than men are surviving to late old age.

In the development of a national policy on ageing, and especially in the effective implementation of a such policy, it is considered that a focal agency or body is vital to initiate and coordinate policies, programmes and projects in all aspects of ageing (ESCAP 2001b). Such an agency is considered advantageous in that it will provide a clear focus and line of responsibility, and could take direct action in a number of programmes. ESCAP did find that the majority (85 per cent) of member states responding to a survey in 2000 reported having a focal agency that was responsible for issues relating to ageing and older persons. However, the functions of such agencies vary, as looking after the welfare of older persons may merely be listed as one of the responsibilities of some government ministries, or the ministry may have established specific divisions or units specifically for older persons. Likewise, with regard to the provision of services for older persons, while it is recommended that this responsibility should lie primarily with governments, support from NGOs and other entities, especially the private sector, is strategic. Close cooperation among all these sectors is regarded as extremely important so, again, the issue of coordination of policies and practice is emphasized.

Key issues and questions addressed

In the light of the issues and various guiding principles discussed above, the authors of the five case-study chapters in this book were invited to address, explicitly or implicitly, a number of key questions in their countries with respect to national policies in general, and those relating to long-term care in particular. These were:

1. Is there an identifiable or less explicit national policy on ageing, or a national policy relating (NPA) to older persons? If so, which ministry or organization takes a lead role in this policy and its coordination? Is there a focal agency?
2. What are the main features of the policy and how long has it been in place? (How comprehensive is it? Which sectors are involved? Is it long-term or short-term? What are the sources of funding, if any?)
3. What is the profile of any NPA: is there a senior politician or administrator responsible for older persons? (In other words, does the policy have any real importance or impact?)
4. If no identifiable policy exists, are there plans or pressures to organize one?
5. Has there been any involvement of civil society, NGOs or older persons themselves in the formulation or development of the policy?
6. In which areas are policy initiatives or major revisions to NPAs likely to be needed in view of demographic and socio-economic trends over the next decade or so?

Key issues in long-term care (LTC)
7. Is there a national policy or strategy on LTC for older persons or, say, on accommodation?
8. Is any policy or strategy headed by a department, ministry or minister?
9. What range of LTC provision exists or is planned?

10. Do policy and practice rely mainly on institutional care, care by families and/or care in the community (is there a blend of sources)?

11. Are there estimates being made and revised of the types and needs of LTC provision (such as numbers of day-care places, respite care, long-and short-stay places, home helpers)?

12. Is there an awareness of the issues surrounding LTC needs and pressures arising from demographic and socio-economic trends? Is there any sense of urgency?

13. Are there any significant obstacles or advantages to the development of LTC (such as heavy reliance on institutional care; excessive reliance on care by family members; and an emphasis of traditional Asian values)?

14. What are the likely future needs and outcomes in LTC provision?

The answers to these questions will be influenced by many explicit and implicit features of the socio-political, health and welfare systems of the individual countries. For example, a policy on ageing or LTC that relies extensively on family care will have a different set of practical, financial and philosophical outcomes and expectations than one that relies heavily on public sector provision. In this respect, the book shows some quite wide-ranging policies. For example, Choi in Chapter 3 indicates how in Korea an entrenched attitude that families will be able to care for their older members, despite the fact that this is an unrealistic expectation, has hindered the development of formal care for older persons and has even made ageing into a national problem. Elsewhere, for example in Singapore, (Mehta, Chapter 5) and Hong Kong (Chan and Phillips, Chapter 2), whilst considerable lip-service is paid to the importance of family care and traditional Asian values such as filial piety (respect and duty of care between parents and children), official statements recognize that families in the modern setting need considerable support if they are to care for older members. Of course, whether such recognition is backed up by services and resources is not always apparent.

The shifting social context: fitter and better-educated older persons in the future?

Policy-makers throughout the Asia–Pacific region, and in the five countries discussed in this book in particular, need to be aware that today's older persons are in many ways an interim generation (Phillips 2000*b*; ESCAP 2001*a*). Future policy must anticipate the emergence of cohorts of older persons in the coming decades who will know and demand their rights, unlike the present generation many of whom are humble and regard the state as the paternalistic authority. Many of tomorrow's older persons will be fitter, better-educated and wealthier. They will expect and demand responsive, high-quality services and provision. Any national policy on ageing that does not take this into account will be fatally flawed. However, a major challenge for the coming decade is likely to be how to develop quality services for future generations whilst dealing today with the needs of poorer and often less healthy people.

The five case-study countries

Through reviewing the development and the current provision of care and services to older people, writers from the five Asian countries or city–states try to pinpoint the strengths and difficulties, as well as to highlight key areas for consideration and improvements in ageing policy and practices. These chapters, for the first time, provide a comprehensive description and analysis of policies on ageing and long-term care, which are the focus of increasing attention and concern within and across societies over the last decade or so. Key features are taken up in detail in the case-study chapters, but first we consider a number of underlying issues that form the background for these chapters.

Demographic ageing of populations

As noted earlier, it is not the intention to discuss demographic data in great detail, but a summary of statistics on population and ageing for the five countries is given in Table 1.1. These data

TABLE 1.1
Demographic Characteristics of the Five Countries, 2001

	Total Population (mid-2001, millions)	Percentage Aged 65+	Sex Ratio[a] Population Aged 60+	Life Expectancy at Birth (ELB)			Dependency Ratio[b]	Total Fertility Rate[c]	Crude Death Rate (per 1000)	Urban Population (%)
				Total	Male	Female				
Hong Kong	6.879	11	94	80	77	82	39	1.0	5.5	100
Korea	47.676	7	72	74	71	78	41	1.5	5.3	82
Malaysia	23.639	4	90	73	70	75	59	3.1	4.4	58
Singapore	4.148	7	87	78	76	80	40	1.5	4.5	100
Thailand	62.968	7	83	72	71	76	49	1.8	6.0	22
ESCAP Region Average	3,781.169	6	85	—	66	69	54	2.5	8.0	38

[a] Males per 100 females.

[b] Dependency ratio: $\dfrac{\text{(population 0–14 + population 65+)}}{\text{population 15–64}} \times 100.$

[c] Average number of children per woman.

Source: ESCAP (2001c).

are drawn principally from the United Nations Economic and Social Commission for Asia and the Pacific *Population Data Sheet 2001* (ESCAP 2001c). The data are therefore presented on a broadly comparable basis. It should be noted that in some of the following chapters, local census updates and other sources have occasionally been used, so that precise matches may not occur with some statistics in Table 1.1.

All five of the case-study countries are facing the rapid growth of an ageing population, although their cut-off ages for defining "older people"are not the same. Indeed, for various purposes internally (retirement ages, pensionable age, granting of certain benefits), individual countries specify different chronological ages. For example, the age requirement for entitlement to elderly services and care in both Thailand and Malaysia is 60 years of age, while in Hong Kong, Korea and Singapore it is 65. Hong Hong and Singapore both have lower retirement ages in some sectors, at 55 (increasing to 60) in Singapore and at 60 in Hong Kong in many companies and the public sector. However, in Hong Kong, access to allowances for older persons starts at a higher age. Definitions aside, the chronological ageing of the population in most countries is obvious: in Hong Kong, 11 per cent of the population is aged 65+; in Singapore, Thailand and Korea it is 7 per cent; and in Malaysia it is 4 per cent — all substantial increases on the previous decades' figures.

The factors underpinning the increases in the ageing populations are similar across the countries — as they are, of course, worldwide. A major reason for this demographic ageing is a very low fertility rate in four out of the five countries. Hong Kong's total fertility rate (TFR), for example, is about the lowest in the world, at 1.0 children per woman, whilst that of Korea and Singapore is 1.5, and Thailand 1.8. Only Malaysia, at 3.1, has a TFR above the natural replacement rate (usually considered to be about 2.1). Added to the very low TFRs and crude birth rates in the region are gradually-increasing lifespans. The life expectancy at birth of males and females in Hong Kong is 77 and 82 years respectively, whilst comparable figures in Singapore are 76 and 80, and in Malaysia, 70 and 75.

There are also quite high elderly dependency ratios in the case-study countries and, whilst dependency rates are not perfect, they are often taken as an indication of potentially increasing burdens both on the economically-active population and on governments and their economies, especially in the health and welfare sectors. It must be emphasized, however, that dependency ratios are often misused or "over-used" by economists and politicians. Their real impact and true significance in any given country and time are very much influenced by factors such as the prevalence of employment amongst older persons, their savings and economic resources, family care and, of course, the health status of the older population. All these factors are changing in the region. Therefore, there is no uniform or unambiguous impact of an increasing elderly dependency ratio, although it is a figure that it is wise to watch in each country (Table 1.1). In many ways, increasing dependency ratios, like increasing life expectancy, are reflections of success in social and economic policies, good health and nutrition, modern welfare services and a good standard of living for the population.

Provision of services and care

In broad terms, services and care for older persons in these countries can be considered under three categories: social security, health care and social services (ESCAP 2001d).

Social security
To ensure the basic needs of older persons that are met, the governments of some Asia–Pacific countries provide direct financial assistance, although this is very limited. For example, Hong Kong has an Old Age Allowance of approximately HK$625 (US$80) per month, as an asset and income-tested benefit for its citizens aged 65 and over, known colloquially as "fruit money" due to its minimal value. It also has a means-tested Comprehensive Social Security Assistance Scheme, starting at HK$2,555 per month for older persons (aged over 60) with some disability, rising to $4,355 (US$325–558) for poorer older people needing nursing care (Chapter 2). Korea likewise aims to

guarantee a minimum living standard for its older adults through its newly-codified 2000 National Basic Livelihood Security Law, which built on the existing public assistance law, and its likewise small "Elder- Respect Pension" (Chapter 3). In many societies, however, means testing of welfare benefits has tended to imbue them with a stigma and there is often evidence that older persons do not claim their entitlements for reasons of pride and a wish for privacy.

On the other hand, some societies emphasize provident fund schemes to provide income security for their retired workers. For example, in Malaysia, formal sector workers participate in a range of government and private sector pension schemes, but these are not compulsory for the self-employed, amongst whom the participation rate is low (Chapter 4). These people will therefore have to rely largely on their own resources in old age. In Singapore, workers after retirement have to rely on the Central Provident Fund, which was established in 1955 (Chapter 5). Korea has four public pension programmes which function as contributory social insurance schemes (Chapter 3). In Hong Kong, a mandatory employment-based contributory scheme (by employees and employers), the Mandatory Provident Fund, was introduced at the end of 2000. However, this covers only those earning above HK$4,000 (US$512) per month, and it has a low ceiling (HK$20,000 and 5 per cent contributions by both parties). It will clearly therefore take many years for employees to build up sufficient funds in their personal MPF accounts to give any financial security in retirement. As in Malaysia, the self-employed and low income earners can slip through the net. Korea has noticed the same problem, and has an old-age allowance, now termed the Elder-Respect Pension, to help those people who were not covered by the national pension scheme of 1988 because they were already of retirement age.

Health care
Health services comprise a wide range of curative and promotive services, at the community (primary care) level, ranging from clinics to increasingly specialized hospitals and institutions. In all the countries covered by this book, in addition to Western-

style allopathic medicine, with mainly a disease-oriented nature, there also exists an important parallel — and sometimes connected — system of traditional Asian medicine. This may be in the form of traditional Chinese doctors, pharmacists, acupuncturists and bone-setters in Hong Kong, Singapore and parts of Malaysia and Thailand, or other forms of Indian and Buddhist medical services in Malaysia, Singapore and Thailand. Older persons often find traditional sources of health care a great comfort and culturally acceptable (Phillips 1990). In the societies in this book, such traditional health care is mainly available only through the private sector.

When in need of formal Western health care and services, older adults, in all the societies under discussion, tend to rely mainly on publicly-provided government facilities, particularly for hospital and rehabilitative services. This is because few older persons have the resources or insurance to pay for private sector Western-style medicine — although there are exceptions, such as people with special coverage, retired armed forces personnel and some civil servants in some countries. By and large, however, the older population will at present rely on out-of-pocket primary care or, if in need of hospital care, they turn to the public sector.

Most countries in this book provide at least basic hospital services for their older populations, even if these are sometimes crowded and difficult to access. Many have already implemented, or at least have plans to introduce, insurance schemes to lessen the financial burden of medical services. Korea, for example, started a medical insurance programme in 1977, and Malaysia has also recently developed such a scheme. Hong Kong does not as yet have any compulsory medical insurance schemes, depending mainly on the private sector to provide insurance programmes for individuals — although this is an area of active debate, partly spurred by the poor economic climate in the region post-1997.

The health status of the current and future cohorts of older persons in the five countries is also very important. At present, as noted above, expectation of life at birth is generally extending and ranges from (male/female) 70/75 years in Malaysia to 77/82 years in Hong Kong. The health status of the older population is apparently improving gradually, although chronic and degenerative conditions are emerging increasingly, such as heart disease, and circulatory and musculo-skeletal disorders. There is no compelling evidence as yet as to whether there is a compression of morbidity in the region (that is, a longer life with a relatively shorter period of ill-health or disability before death) or longer life and worsening health status. This is clearly a very important question for policy-makers, and it will underpin decisions about the sorts of community and institutional services that are needed. Indeed, it will influence the nature of the medical and nursing skills and the training needed in the future, as well as many other issues. As a result, research needs to be conducted and epidemiological data systematically gathered as soon as possible.

The continuing good health of younger generations can impact on older persons in a number of ways if they are expected to be earners and carers. A specific issue may occur in some countries of the region where there is likely to be an impact from the morbidity and mortality of intermediate generations, for example from HIV/Aids which is likely to significantly affect Thailand, Burma (Myanmar), the Philippines and perhaps China (HelpAge International 2002). As Gorman (1999) has noted, the most unfortunate older people can be those who live utterly alone or with young, dependent grandchildren yet with no middle generation. Such a scenario is unfortunately increasingly common in some African countries and may appear in the Asia–Pacific (Knodel et al. 2001).

Social services
The third category of services, social services, involves provision of services and assistance in kind, as well as housing or specialist accommodation for older persons. The range and depth of services developed in the five Asia–Pacific countries under discussion are varied according to their different contextual needs. Some social services, such as recreational services, are generic and serve all ages, whilst others are more focused on older persons and include those such as institutional care, day care, personal care and home-help services. Issues related to the status and morale of older persons are sometimes also covered, and can include promoting

the employment of older persons. Unlike the other countries, Korea and Singapore increasingly emphasize elderly employment, Singapore in part because of predicted potential labour shortages.

The need for specialist or adapted forms of accommodation to enable some older persons to continue living in the community and to avoid institutionalization is widely recognized (see, for example, Heumann and Boldy 1993; Phillips and Yeh 1999). Therefore, given the nature of demographic ageing in the countries in this book, with large percentage increases expected in the numbers of older persons, coupled with social changes which are diminishing family care abilities, it is not surprising that housing forms a major plank in most social services/welfare policies. All of the following chapters consider the ranges of accommodation available and policies relating to housing in the case-study countries. These range from policies to promote "ageing in place" (ageing *in situ*) and community care, to the provision of long-stay residential and hospital units with day-round nursing care. Home care and associated support is clearly crucial in this (Mende 2001). Some countries — such as Singapore and Hong Kong — with their large quasi-public housing provision, specifically aim part of their housing policy for older persons at strategies to enable families to keep living with or near elderly relatives. These strategies include allocation of housing units (apartments) nearby for children and elderly parents, and more rapid allocation of public housing when older relatives are included. It is strongly predicted that these types of initiatives will gain in importance in the region, as the public sector tries to maintain family care and co-residence or residence nearby of older people and their younger relatives, and to foster "traditional Asian values" such as filial piety (Ng et al. 2002). In addition, policies to enable unrelated older persons to live together are also being attempted and may well expand as widowhood and longevity increase.

The philosophical bases to and nature of national ageing policies

National policies on ageing are developed in a complex set of contexts: socio-cultural, political, economic and international. The international context in particular is becoming increasingly important in the region, as research and knowledge, of the types of services and provision for older persons that exist in different parts of the world become known. Also very important is the socio-cultural context, as all the countries in the region — one can say ubiquitously — regard older persons with traditional respect and love, even if this is not always translated into care and resources. The family is also widely regarded as the main and acceptable — indeed, expected — provider of care and financial support. This is both a strength and a weakness in the development of national policies on ageing, as many of the authors in this book echo.

Although the details of care and services provisions are different among the five case-study countries, the nature and philosophy reflected in their implementation are in many ways more or less similar in all. This fact offers some insights which may be useful for planning and improving the policies and care for ageing populations in the region.

Although the growth of the ageing population, and the need for policies with a longer-term perspective, is apparent, not all countries have a clear policy on ageing. Thailand did not have formal national policies on ageing until 1986 and Malaysia until 1995. Singapore's policies have been formatted even more recently, but an impressive integration is rapidly developing, at least at the inter-ministerial level of the government and including prominent NGOs. Singapore's Inter-Ministerial Committee on the Ageing Population was set up in 1998 to propose a coordinated and comprehensive approach, following a review of the health care needs of older persons (Inter-Ministerial Committee on the Ageing Population 1999; Inter-Ministerial Committee on Health Care for the Elderly 1999). Hong Kong and Korea do not as yet have a central policy framework focusing on their older citizens, although both are working towards this goal. Since 1997, Hong Kong has established an Elderly Commission as a type of umbrella organization that coordinates major policies on health, welfare and housing. However, government departments and some NGOs still tend to pursue their own agendas, although many are now becoming more focused and coordinated.

All the chapters point out that a principal aim of policies on ageing (however well formulated) in the five countries is to keep older people in the community for as long as possible. This, as noted earlier, is often referred to as "ageing in place" and is accompanied by a range of community care philosophies and initiatives, some of which are effective, others less so. For example, the Hong Kong Special Administrative Region Government encourages "ageing in place" and "community care", while Singapore promotes social integration and integrated delivery of care services at the community level. A major outcome of this orientation is a belated recognition of the importance of home support and community care services.

Top-down approaches
It is also important to identify the pervasive role of the state in the five case studies, which extends in many from the economic sphere to those of the social and demographic. Today, and in the recent past, the welfare policies for older persons that have operated in these countries have been very much government-led. Whilst lip-service has been paid to consumer demand, the voices of older persons themselves have been relatively muted in most countries, although today older people's action groups are increasingly vocal (although not to the extent that this is seen in North America, Europe and Australia–New Zealand). Singapore uses "supply-side socialism" as a welfare strategy to avoid abuse by the recipient, while Korea has maintained the principle of "economic growth then distribution". Hong Kong has very much been a benevolent dictatorship in welfare policy terms , although this may change as economic and political pressures mount in the SAR.

Unanimously, the five case studies recognize the importance of the family (however defined) in care for older people, particularly long-term care and financial support. These still depend greatly on family and the informal sector in all five countries; the governments of these countries, whilst setting the scene, are the last resort provider of care at the moment, although this is clearly changing. The traditional Asian value of "filial piety" (in Chinese, *xiao*), a two-way duty of care and responsibility between parents and children, is emphasized, especially among the Chinese societies in the region. It also has strong echoes in Korea and amongst the peoples of Thailand and Malaysia. This assumes that older people will be cared for by families and communities, which is encouraged and promoted as the norm of the society. The family is seen as the key caring unit of society and in some countries this has been embodied in law — for example, in Singapore, in the Maintenance of Parents Act (1995).

This reliance on family care is a great strength and something of which these societies may justifiably be proud. However, its uncritical acceptance and, more importantly, the continuing expectation that families in the twenty-first century will be able to continue their functions as carers for older persons has been identified as a potential weakness (Choi 2000a; Phillips 2000b; Ng et al 2002). This is particularly so when children are made to feel guilty if they are not able to take full care of their parents, however old or frail, and when their own domestic and economic circumstances make such care difficult. In Korea, the unbending expectation that families will be the primary care-givers has been seen to have actually deterred the development of coherent policies and effective public services for older persons (Chapter 3). As a result, there is now growing pressure within Korean society for these expectations to be amended. In Hong Kong, the chief executive, Tung Chee-Wah, has explicitly stated that there must be services and other forms of assistance available, so that families can continue to shoulder what may become an increasingly heavy burden if left to themselves. Similar sentiments are echoed in Singapore and Thailand, and Malaysia is also starting to recognize this issue, although the country faces slightly less demographic pressure than the others at present.

Whilst families undoubtedly do still have a very important caring function in all the countries under discussion, the ability of older persons to choose where they would like to live and with whom is also important. This will grow with future older cohorts, who will be better-educated and better off than many of today's older persons. If asked where they would like to live, many older persons state "with their children", but this is an ideal. In reality, many older persons prefer their independence, and for personal reasons do not actually want to live with their children and risk inter-generational conflicts.

A number of practical factors militate against the family's easy continuation of care. First, many families are split by migration for work and because of social issues such as bereavement or divorce. Second, family sizes are decreasing and will be even smaller in the future, reducing the numbers of children to share the social and economic responsibilities of care for elderly parents. The combined effects of these two factors mean that many future older persons may not have any children living nearby on whom they can rely. Third, housing space is at a premium and, in most Asian cities, dwellings large enough to accommodate multi-generations are becoming rarer and very expensive. Fourth, economic circumstances and social choice mean that many more women, the traditional carers for elderly parents or parents-in-law, are working and are not available as constant free carers. Last but not least, as noted above, many older persons themselves would prefer the freedom to live independently, if perhaps near to their children and grandchildren. This aspect, the welfare of older persons, is very important. Many do not wish to live in the same house as their children and do not wish to be perceived as burdens on them, especially in hard economic times.

All these factors operate in various combinations in the countries covered by the book. They heavily underscore the urgent need for policies and provision to be developed that will help families and will not place crushing burdens on them. The family as a caring institution is a resource and needs nurturing and supporting.

Problems and prospects

The case studies in this book provide detailed information in the wide arena of general national policies on ageing and the related area of long-term care. Some problems have been highlighted, but the picture is not wholly gloomy as there are also considerable grounds for optimism. The authors of all five case studies identify the need for coherent planning and the urgency of action for long-term care to deal with the increasing ageing population and currently limited provision of care and services. All authors implicitly and explicitly recognize the challenges of developing policies and services for today's cohorts of older persons. As noted above, in many ways they are an "interim generation", few of whom have personal financial resources or pensions, and who still may want traditional family support. The future generations in the region will be fitter and better educated, as well as being more financially secure — at least amongst those in the urban formal sector.

At present, most authors find that current policies for and implementation of services to older people tend to be fragmented, but most also note that changes are now under way. In many countries, a "focal agency" is in existence, but it may at times view its remit too narrowly or may not be of a sufficiently high political profile to be able to effect changes. Coordination is another issue that some governments have tackled head on, as in Singapore's inter-ministerial committees, whilst elsewhere, it is still being grappled with. In Hong Kong, for example, there are three main executive departments (the Hospital Authority, the Department of Health and the Social Welfare Department) responsible for different services for older persons. A problem with this system is a lack of coordination in service delivery across these departments as well as with the private sector and NGOs. Therefore, integration and coordination within and across different institutions and sectors is essential, and it is hoped that the Elderly Commission established in 1997 will have enough power to achieve this. Singapore has addressed a similar phenomenon, and has in the past signalled a wish to develop coordinated inter-sectoral policies through high-profile inter-ministerial committees, especially in the late 1990s.

Whilst national policies on ageing are developing and are manifestly needed in the region, they are generally still at a fairly nascent stage of development (Howe and Phillips 2001). However, across the region as a whole there is clearly a great deal of activity going on, and the future looks quite optimistic (ESCAP 2001*a* and 2001*b*). Clearly, too, a number of specific issues remain to be dealt with in many countries; the provision and affordability of care and services to older people, and their availability, accessibility and affordability, are the main concerns, regardless of contextual differences among the countries. Adequacy and availability issues are highlighted in many chapters — for example, an inadequacy of community-based services in Thailand and Malaysia, and a shortage of appropriate health services in Hong Kong, Singapore and Korea. Three of the countries have an additional and common phenomenon to address: the imbalance in the distribution of services across urban and rural areas, which is particularly problematic in Malaysia and is also evident in Thailand and Korea.

Long-term care also needs to be looked at within the broad context of the types of accommodation available and the likely personnel availability for community support, and also in terms of the characteristics of future elderly cohorts. In this respect, the feminization of ageing is noted in all the case studies. Well over half of the elderly population will be female, which often means long periods of widowhood, potentially with reduced economic resources (Lee 2001a). Such considerations will need to inform planning for policies on ageing and long-term care in the future. The planning of the types of staff required, skill levels and skill mixes, and the amount of support that will be available must all be carefully considered as the following chapters suggest. National policies on ageing and on long-term care must recognize the needs for training of sufficient personnel, so syllabus setting and standards become crucial. Within services themselves, the public sector has a heavy responsibility for standard-setting and regulation, and the concomitant inspection to maintain such standards. The implementation of inspection can be, if desired, by independent public sector inspectors, or it can be a private sector function. However, governments must ultimately be responsible for the setting of standards and for following up when quality is not sufficient.

2

Policies on Ageing and Long-term Care in Hong Kong

Alfred C. M. Chan & David R. Phillips

Introduction

It is an issue of debate whether an policy on ageing currently
exists or has ever existed in Hong Kong. Formal government
concern for older persons' welfare started in the early 1970s,
when the growing population of older persons began to stir official
interest in formulating a policy for the welfare of the elderly in
general and needy older persons in particular. Such interest has
progressed intermittently over the subsequent three decades,
although a comprehensive and applied policy is still to emerge.

Indeed, if "policy" is taken to mean a coherent conceptual
framework linking different practices for the achievement of a
goal or mission, the gradual development of such a policy
framework has been evident since the 1970s, but services provided
have not always been consistent with the policy. However, if
"policy" is taken more generally and pragmatically to imply a
central government effort towards collating public services, then
there has been, at the most, only a direction for formulating such
policy. In the 1970s, there was no evidence of a central policy

framework. Using the first conceptual framework for the present review, the government of the Hong Kong started looking at ageing issues in the 1970s, and actually made a number of attempts to formulate a central policy in the 1980s and 1990s. However, coordination between the different service departments became so difficult that issues related to ageing became focused principally on health and personal social service issues, the policy responsibility for which lies with the Health and Welfare Bureau. Things have changed somewhat since Mr Tung Chee-hwa became chief executive of the Hong Kong Special Administrative Region (HKSAR) of China, as it has been termed since 1 July 1997. After his first-term election in 1997 (he was re-elected in 2002), Mr Tung announced that three commissions would be set up to attempt an overview of their respective areas: the Housing Commission, the Education Commission and the Elderly Commission. Whilst these commissions have no executive power, they do play a key consultative role in policy-making.

Today, what might be called the present policy on ageing in Hong Kong essentially reflects the efforts of the chief executive and one of his policy units, the Health and Welfare Bureau (HWB), which is responsible for policies related to health and personal social service. The Elderly Commission (EC), formed in late 1997 with the chief executive's blessing, essentially plays an advisory and consultative role, or at least a coordinating role. Perhaps its major impact has been to give at least the semblance of an overview and discussion forum/think tank, in which disparate and rather uncoordinated departments and agencies concerned with issues relating to older persons are forced to meet and interact. Policy initiatives developed so far have mainly been in the provision of guidelines for three principal executive departments — the Hospital Authority (HA), responsible for hospital treatment and rehabilitation, the Department of Health, responsible for health promotion and disease prevention, and the Social Welfare Department, responsible for personal social services. Other departments, acting largely on their own initiative, have implemented complementary policy to improve services for older persons.

For example, the Housing Bureau and the Housing Authority have cooperated with the EC and the HWB to develop specially designed housing packages for elderly people and their families. At the present, therefore, a national policy on ageing is still effectively at the stage of formulation, although there are several initiatives for drawing up a more coherent policy.

This chapter highlights the evolution and probable future direction of policy development in the provision of services for elderly people in Hong Kong. Despite the promulgation of its first White Paper on ageing and service in 1973, and the subsequent 1976 government Programme Plan on services for the elderly, these early worthy initiatives largely failed because the government could not implement them, mainly due to the poor economic conditions prevailing at the time. However, as the economy grew strongly in the 1980s, spending on elderly services became ever more generous. Today and in the future, increasing resources are likely to be required in the light of the demographically ageing population and the increasing costs of providing health and social care services. This has prompted the HKSAR Government to look at cost savings through what has been termed its Enhanced Productivity Programme, which looks for better ways of serving the elderly population (among others) and boosting and conserving revenue. A controversy arose in 2000–01 over the introduction of a Mandatory Provident Fund for retirement saving and protection, as well as some suggestions to introduce compulsory contributions for long-term care, possibly among those aged over 40. These have both been controversial because of the historical lack of any compulsory territory-wide retirement savings scheme and the fact that, for the previous decade or more, Hong Kong residents had enjoyed health and social care almost free of charge. To now ask them to pay at the start of the new century is a challenge for the administration. These financial issues are of growing importance in elderly service planning as in other sectors, and even more so for long-term care, as discussed below.

It is important to be aware that, as in most sectors in the Hong Kong administration, policy-making in welfare, in general, is government-led. Private sector hospital capacity is very limited. Although over 95 per cent of personal social services are run by NGOs and almost all hospital services are run by the Hospital Authority (an independently-governed public organization), government executives dominate policy-making through a substantial public funding mechanism known locally as "subvention". This subvention to date has guaranteed these organizations full subsidies, year after year, as long as their practices meet government-set standards. There is therefore little scope or incentive for variation in service provision by districts or by the various organizations involved.

The historical and demographic background to development of policy on ageing

Hong Kong was a British colony from 1841 until 1 July 1997, when sovereignty reverted to China. Until 1997, policy-making was characterized by many features of colonialism tempered by the imperative to safeguard economic growth, and was often reactionary and remedial. For most important issues, approval and endorsement rested with the governor, the appointed administration and, ultimately, with the government in Britain, which generally had little interest in day-to-day welfare issues. Many commentators feel that it is arguable whether things have really changed much since 1997, with Beijing exhibiting a similar, if geographically closer, benevolent neglect with regard to welfare issues. The most obvious differences are the appointment of a Chinese chief executive (Mr Tung Chee-hwa), a new Court of Final Appeal, and the enactment of the Basic Law, which governs the Hong Kong SAR and its relations with China and the world. Most senior civil servants, including the heads of policy units and service-provider departments, have in general continued to serve the SAR government since the handover of sovereignty. At least on the surface, the machinery for policy-making has continued almost seamlessly without significant changes.

Rapid demographic ageing

As in much of the region, it is not easy in Hong Kong to define who is "elderly". There exists a local tradition that someone aged 60 or above is taken to be an elderly person — and many organizations, including the government, regard this as retirement age — but the picture is variable. For example, some public organizations have 65 as the qualifying age for free or subsidized services, such as social security payments, medical and health services, so there is a gap of five years between what different agencies consider to be the target groups for elderly policy-making. Bearing this in mind, the present chapter adopts the internationally fairly widely accepted age of 65 as the chronological cut-off defining "old age" in policy terms.

The demographic ageing of Hong Kong's population first became particularly noticeable in the early 1970s, constituting then 4.5 per cent to 6.6 per cent of the total population (Phillips 1988a, 1992). The growth continued with roughly 1 per cent for each of the five years to the present, with people aged 65 and above accounting for 11.1 per cent of the total population in the year 2001 (see Table 2.1, Table 2.2 and Figure 2.1).

Like many other countries in the region, Hong Kong's rapidly growing ageing population, as well as advances in

TABLE 2.1

Hong Kong: Growth of the Population Aged 65 and Above, 1971–2016

Year	Number	Percentage of Total Population
1971	178,000	4.5
1976	243,000	5.5
1981	327,000	6.6
1986	409,000	7.6
1991	482,000	8.7
1996	630,000	10.0
2001	747,000	11.1
2016[a]	—	13.0

[a] Estimate

Source: Census and Statistics Department, Hong Kong (1997, 2002a).

TABLE 2.2

Hong Kong: Mid-year Population by Age Group

Age Group	1995 (mid-year) ('000)	%	1999 (mid-year) ('000)	%	2001 (Census) ('000)	%
Under 15	1,195.1	19.4	1,182.9	17.6	1,109.4	16.5
15–64	4,359.2	70.8	4,802.9	71.5	4,851.9	72.3
65 and over	601.8	9.8	734.9	10.9	747.1	11.1
Total	6,156.1	100.0	6,720.7	100.0	6,708.4	100.0

Source: Census and Statistics Department, Hong Kong (1996, 1997, 2002*a*).

FIGURE 2.1

Hong Kong: Population Projections, 1997–2016

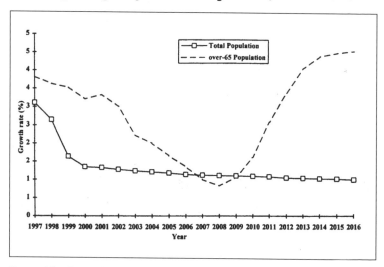

Source: After Liu and Wong (1997).

lifestyles and environmental and health provisions, which tend to lengthen life expectancy (Table 2.3) , have generally increased the size of the "dependent" population (Table 2.4). This can suggest the need for a whole range of public services, including long-term care.

TABLE 2.3
Hong Kong: Expectation of Life at Selected Ages, 1977–2016

	Age			
	Male		Female	
Year	*At birth*	*At 60*	*At birth*	*At 60*
1977	70.1	16.4	76.7	21.1
1986	74.1	18.5	79.4	22.6
1996	76.3	20.0	81.8	24.1
2006[a]	77.5	20.8	82.8	24.8
2016[a]	78.1	21.1	83.4	25.1

[a] 2006 and 2016 figures are projections.
Source: Census and Statistics Department, Hong Kong (1997).

TABLE 2.4
Hong Kong: Elderly Dependency Ratios, 1997–2016

Year	Number of Elderly Aged 65+ (*a*)	Number of Persons Aged 15–64 ('000) (*b*)	Elderly Dependency Ratio (*a* ÷ *b*)
1977	261,100	2,993.1	87.2
1986	423,700	3,826.9	110.8
1996	631,300	4,471.8	141.2
2001	753,600	4,867.2	154.8
2006[a]	830,200	5,411.2	153.4
2016[a]	1,091,700	5,926.8	184.2

[a] Figures for 2006 and 2016 are projected figures only.
Sources: Census and Statistics Department, Hong Kong (1996, 1997, 2002*b*).

Living arrangements can be a significant indicator of levels of direct family support in Hong Kong. Census data indicate that, in 1996 and 2001, about 10 per cent of people aged 60 and over lived alone and 67 per cent lived with another family member, either a spouse, a child or a sibling. Income levels of older persons are also generally poor. In 1996, for example,

67 per cent (59,438) of people aged 60 and above had an income below the local social security cut-off level of approximately US$250 per month. However, data disaggregated by age groups have been generally lacking and information can only be assessed via non-census sources, such as research projects by tertiary institutes and individual researchers in Hong Kong. This is a weakness in policy terms, as data on topics such as the prevalence in the community of chronic illness, disability, income sources and social support are vital for accurate policy-making.

Meeting the major needs of the ageing population: housing, health and social services

The various former colonial governments' responses to the increasing number of older persons were simple: to create services for needs identified by professionals and relevant government departments. An policy on ageing as such was not deemed necessary to coordinate all services to meet these needs, and a "first come first served", approach meant that service developments were effectively a product of economic growth and ad hoc initiatives from sympathetic departments. In broad terms, the 1970s may be viewed as a period of acknowledging demands identified by professionals, but the government did not have the resources to do much in practical terms. However, the 1980s was a boom period for elderly services as a result of a high budget surpluses. The 1990s was a period of consolidation and contraction, as the economy began to falter. Throughout this period, especially 1997 to 2000, a more elderly-focused, yet service-led rather than charity-led, model of service provision emerged. The relevant departments concerned — predominantly the Social Welfare Department (SWD) and Medical and Health Services, now split into the Hospital Authority (HA) and the Department of Health (DH), and the Housing Authority — started modifying their services to focus on the elderly as a distinct user group. Services were generally confined to the departmental level rather than efforts being cross-departmental or inter-sectoral. Service types, though broadly covered, were therefore not particularly well integrated and coordinated. It is against this background that the present service provision may be viewed, in line with the socio-economic, physical, and psychological status of the present ageing population.

Housing services and schemes

Housing services in Hong Kong are provided by quasi-independent authorities such as the Hong Kong Housing Authority, which is responsible mainly for public housing development, and the Hong Kong Housing Society, a non-profit-making organization which is essentially self-financing. The housing and accommodation needs of the elderly population have been shaped mainly by a number of social trends. These include a growing demand for separate living (principally from children), an increasing desire for privacy and a disinclination for multi-generational sharing, especially given the small size of housing units (mainly apartments) that predominate in Hong Kong. Very high housing costs, however, are a major factor that can sometimes cause families to share, even if unwillingly. Newly-designed units have taken these various demands into consideration, and a review of the earlier evolution of housing for older persons may be seen in Phillips (1988*b*).

The 1997 General Household Survey showed that, of a total 920,000 people aged 60 and above, some 416,400 lived in public housing estates maintained by the Housing Authority and Housing Society; 92,500 were in government subsidized home-ownership schemes; and the remaining 411,500 were in other private accommodation or in institutions such as nursing homes and hospitals. In general, public housing units are in strong demand in Hong Kong due to low rentals, and many applicants, even though they may satisfy residence and income criteria, have to wait for more than six years to be allocated a place. Older persons have been accorded priority in housing allocation through a variety of schemes, but the average waiting time for a single unit is still about four years. The demand ratio set for public housing units for the elderly was estimated to be 54 per cent in 1997. However, in view of the rapid increase in demand for single units by older persons, as well as the discovery of a substantial number of people residing in residential homes who ought to be in ordinary housing units (Deloitte and Touche 1997), the demand ratio has been increased to 60 per cent. This is to cope with the projected population aged 60 and above of 1,126,300 elderly people by 2006–07, and to avoid people inappropriately occupying residential care for housing needs. A variety of housing schemes have been established to help accommodate older persons, some of which aim to encourage older persons to live with their families — a popular if somewhat misplaced concept in Hong Kong and similar societies. The major schemes are as follows:

The single elderly priority housing scheme.   This scheme has been operating since 1985. The normal waiting period is about four years for a single unit and about two years for elderly group homes. There are about 11,500 elderly people living in such units in public housing estates.

Priority housing scheme for two applicants.   Under this scheme, any two older persons, related or unrelated and who are willing to live together in a two-person unit, can be allocated accommodation within two years. There are about 14,400 people living in such units.

Elderly in family priority scheme.   For families willing to live with one or more of their elderly relatives, the waiting period for public housing will be reduced to three years. Some 13,000 families have been housed under this scheme.

On the face of it, housing provision for older persons in Hong Kong seems well organized, although sufficient capacity is a challenge. However, housing design in general has been geared to people who are capable of looking after themselves rather than for frail or disabled persons. To address these needs, new initiatives are emerging that will incorporate "universal design" concepts in new housing units.

Health services

Government-maintained health services are the responsibility principally of the Department of Health (DH) and the Hospital Authority (HA). The DH takes care of primary health care areas, including environmental hygiene, health promotion, disease prevention and general out-patient clinics (although general practitioners in Hong Kong are private operators who work outside the government scheme and who often offer their services in an uncoordinated manner). The HA looks after hospital and rehabilitative services. The private sector accounts for over 90 per cent of clinic and out-patient services yet for fewer than 10 per cent of hospital beds (Tung 2000). For older persons, mainly those of a lower social status, government-maintained health services are the main source of support.

Primary health care services
Primary health care should provide accessible care, at a local level, to maintain health and reduce morbidity. This is the first level of care, and it is especially important for older persons (Phillips 2000b). In Hong Kong, older persons are being urged to improve their eating habits and to exercise more to achieve "healthy living", which is a slogan and policy of the HA. The message for older persons in Hong Kong is clear: be active, eat well and quit smoking. They are encouraged to engage in physical activities that may enhance endurance and reduce the risk of many potentially fatal diseases, such as coronary heart disease and respiratory diseases, as well of osteoporosis.

In addressing the health care needs of older persons, the DH operates 12 elderly health centres which promote health education and screen individuals as a preventative measure. Similar programmes are also occasionally run by out-patient clinics and non-governmental organizations (NGOs).

Dental health care is an area of considerable weakness in preventative health care, as it focuses on dental health education and prevention rather than on curative treatment. Hong Kong's elderly people are well below the world average in dental care, and in recent years the University of Hong Kong Dental School has been running out-reach services using dental students to assess and attend to older persons. According to World Health Organization (WHO) data, 10 per cent of Hong Kong's elderly people have no teeth (WHO expects less than 5 per cent), and 40 per cent have only 20 normal teeth (WHO aims for more than 75 per cent) (Liu and Wong 1997). This is clearly an area that should be of health policy concern, as poor dental health can lead to bad nutrition in older persons and concomitantly poorer overall health status.

The increase in non-communicable and chronic diseases has also been remarkable in the period since 1960 (Phillips 1988a, 2000b). Some three-quarters of Hong Kong's older people are suffering from one or more chronic illnesses; about 48 per cent have high blood pressure and 40 per cent have arthritis. Among the general population, increasing numbers (some 77 per cent), including older persons, are dying of diseases such as cancer and circulatory and respiratory disorders (Elderly Commission Hong Kong 2001).

Curative and rehabilitative services

Curative and rehabilitative services in Hong Kong are provided by both the public and private sectors, with the private sector providing about 85 per cent of general out-patient services but only 8 per cent of hospital services. The main reason for this pattern is pricing. Out-patient charges for government-maintained clinics are US$5, which includes medication and examination, while private clinics charge about US$20 just for a consultation. The cost of beds in private-sector hospitals can be very high, while the HA hospitals charge only US$8 per day, which includes food and treatment. Public clinics and hospitals also are accessible to all, and would attract yet more people if the services provided were to improve. Currently, they are heavily utilized and waiting times for routine procedures or non-emergency surgery are lengthy.

Currently, out-patient clinics are run by the DH but will ultimately come under the HA for better service integration between clinics and hospitals. There are 68 clinics in Hong Kong and the outlying islands. In the less accessible areas, mobile clinics have been set up. Older people aged 65 and over constitute over

34 per cent of the total out-patients for general consultations (Liu and Wong 1997). Heavy demands are placed on clinic services. A clinic normally sets a daily (Monday to Friday) quota of about 200 consultations, on a "first come, first served" basis. Elderly patients can phone for an appointment, but it is not guaranteed that they can see a doctor. The normal practice for many older persons is therefore to queue up from about 5 or 6 a.m., to wait for an average of four hours before being seen by a doctor. Specialist clinics are attached to hospitals and the demand is similar to that for general out-patient services. On average, there is a three-month wait to see a specialist and, for non-emergency surgery, the waiting time in 2001 was a minimum of nine months.

Community health services aim to maintain older persons at home for as long as possible, in line with the "care in the community "and "ageing in place" philosophies in Hong Kong. A range of services is available, including community geriatric and psycho-geriatric assessment teams (CGATs or PGTs), community nursing services (CNS, both general and psychiatric) and day hospitals. CGATs and PGTs are multi-disciplinary teams conducting regular out-reach services in centres for the elderly and private nursing homes. Their main task is to make accurate assessment of the needs of elderly people and to provide the necessary medical and health support. In 2001, there were 10 CGATs serving about 16,500 patients a year, and 9 PGTs serving about 42,000 patients a year. Of patients served by CNS, 55 per cent were aged 65 and over. Services commonly rendered are injections for diabetes, wound cleansing and continence maintenance. There were 415 day hospital beds serving 93,400 patients in 1998, with an equivalent of 225 patients for each bed, reflecting a grave shortage of such hospital beds.

In 1997, it was estimated that about 20 per cent of Hong Kong's elderly population had at least one form of physical disability and about 50 per cent had at least one chronic illness (Liu and Wong, 1997). Such people are frequent users of hospitals. Indeed, 45 per cent of the current hospital population comprises patients aged 65 or over, who have an average stay of 22 days — 50 per cent longer than the mean.

There are obvious shortfalls in health services for older persons in Hong Kong early in the twenty-first century, but there has not been any systematic collation of epidemiological data to underpin a coordinated policy for their needs. Although more provision has been made, it is still not enough to meet public demand. For example, acute-care hospital beds specially for elderly patients increased by around 80 per cent between 1993 and 1998, from 967 to 1,768 beds. Other health care problems identified are a lack of coordination within and between departments. Services within hospitals may be comprehensive, but are often organized in such a bureaucratic manner that referral from one service to another, and the transfer of medical records from one hospital to another, becomes very cumbersome. The gap between health and community-support services is likewise wide. The lack of proper planning in the admission and discharge of patients reflects the poor communication between the parties involved in the care and welfare of older persons in Hong Kong.

Social work (personal social services)

Social work services in Hong Kong are the responsibility of the Social Welfare Department (SWD) and have two main components: the administration and delivery of social security payments and intervention in personal and social problems. The former function is a direct service rendered by the SWD, while most (over 99 per cent) of the latter function has been rendered through publicly-subvented NGOs.

Social security

The present cohort of older persons is characterized by low literacy, low savings and a lack of sufficient retirement pensions. A relatively large proportion (15 per cent) of the elderly population claims social security benefits, and a report by Oxfam and the Hong Kong Council of Social Service in 1995 claimed that the poverty figures (those receiving or having an income below social security payments threshold) might actually be under-reported. The report argues that many older persons simply do not claim benefits and would rather survive on minimal incomes, even resorting to picking through garbage. The benefits received by older persons include Old Age Allowance (OAA, in 2002 valued at about US$80 per month, means-tested), Comprehensive Social Security Allowance (CSSA, about US$325 per month, means tested) and Disability Allowances (comprising higher CSSA rates) (Lee 2001*b*; and <www.info.gov.hk/swd>). These amounts are believed to be at subsistence level and exclude social expenses that could add to an older person's quality of life. Nonetheless, the annual costs to public expenditure of providing social security payments for older persons totals HK$4–5 billion (US$1 = HK$7.8).

Personal social services

Given Hong Kong's history, it is not surprising that the type and organization of personal social services in Hong Kong broadly follows the British model. Statutory services are the responsibility of the SWD. Other case-work and non-statutory services (comprising over 90 per cent of the total) are delivered principally by NGOs under government subventions administered by the SWD that cover 70 to 100 per cent of costs.

Services to older persons have been developed on the basis of a healthy–frailty continuum. Social centres for the elderly (SEs) cater for people able to lead an independent life. Activities in these centres are mainly social and recreational, offered on a membership basis, with about 300–400 members in each centre, each of whom pays a nominal annual registration fee of US$2.60. There are 214 (212 subvented) SEs, each serving a nominal population of about 20,000. A scheme was launched recently to extend SE services to elderly people of poorer health status, and to offer what may be called life-long learning initiatives (such as classes on literacy and personal interests).

The multi-services centres for the elderly (MEs) run several units under one roof: SEs, counselling services, family-life education, volunteer matching and home help. There are some 34 MEs, each serving a population of 200,000 and with about 2,000 members. Counselling services have been mainly case-work type services while family-life education normally operates mass community education programmes to promote healthy living and intergenerational relationships. Volunteer matching is an attempt to match older people in good health with frail persons, so that healthy volunteers can regularly visit their more frail friends. Home-help services include meals-on-wheels, assistance with household chores and escorts to local clinics for less-able elderly people living at home.

Day-care centres for the elderly (DEs) principally provide services for older persons who are frail yet still able to live at home if they have support. Services include personal and nursing care such as baths, wound dressing, medication and simple exercises to maintain mobility. There are some 38 DEs (34 subvented), each catering to a population of 200,000 and serving a maximum of 40 members at any one time.

There is a plan to integrate these three types of centres into a district-based centre for the elderly, on the basis that different services would be better coordinated and utilized for needy people under one structure. As "ageing in place" and a "community care" philosophies become the guiding policy principles for the development of services for older persons in Hong Kong, there are conscious moves to re-engineer these centre-based services. The new model is to offer an out-reach component, with services targeted to frail older persons confined at home, which will enhance home-care packages.

Nevertheless, there are recognized limitations to "care in the community " . It sometimes becomes necessary for older persons to live in an institution, and for this there is a range of residential choice. Hostels and homes for the aged are designed for able older persons who need just a bed in the former and some limited supervision in the latter. There is a section in homes for the aged for people who need meals cooked and clothes washed for them. A recent move by the SWD was to focus on the really frail people in residential care and to encourage the more able to live in their own homes. Hence, hostels and homes for the aged will fade out while emphasis is placed on care and attention (C&A) homes and nursing homes (NH) for frail persons who need various amounts of C&A and nursing care. There are 193 subvented and self-financed homes providing some 22,000 beds. The private sector provides over 50 per cent of all C&A and NH capacity, some 25,000 places in over 500 homes. The demand for C&A and NH places has been huge, with about 20,000 people on the waiting list at the end of the year 2001. The public reliance on the private sector has inexorably led to legislation to regulate the quality and conduct of these homes. Indeed the regulation of all nursing homes is now governed by the Residential Care Homes (Elderly Persons) Ordinance, enacted in 1994, partially enforced in 1995 and fully implemented in 1996. The ordinance gives the director of the Social Welfare Department the authority for licensing all homes for the elderly in Hong Kong.

Hong Kong therefore today has a fairly comprehensive range of health and social care services for older persons. These are generally easily accessible and, private homes apart, are almost free or low-cost at the point of delivery. However, capacity limitations and the quality of some residential homes, especially in the private sector, are still a matter of concern. Health services can even be considered as universal, as they are heavily subsidized and can be used by anyone. However, in policy terms, there is still a lack of evidence-based policy-making and of coordination in service delivery. In order to understand why this is so, a review of the emergence of the pioneering elderly policy and its development is necessary.

Policy on ageing from the 1970s to 2000

The first Programme Plan for the Elderly was drawn up by the Social Services Branch of the Government Secretariat in September 1977, around the date at which the government began to appreciate the special needs of older persons. The plan went so far as to indicate the inadequacies of services provided for the elderly population in general and also to identify the need for policy and service coordination among government departments and between service providers. The plan acknowledged that many elderly people were in high-risk groups, taking into consideration the usual at-risk population indicators such as living alone, overcrowding, sharing basic facilities, chronic illnesses and/or disability. In June 1982, a five-year review of the plan was issued, with the Central Coordinating Committee on Services to the

Elderly in the Social Services Branch of the Government Secretariat responsible for follow-up reviews. Major features of the 1982 plan included:

- an acknowledgement of the increase in the elderly population, with projections of Hong Kong becoming an ageing society
- details of the possible problems faced by older persons at risk, although the plan did not reveal the causes and extent of the problems
- Suggestions for new, separate services, specially designed for older persons

Social services for the elderly were then organized as separate services, managed mainly by the Social Welfare Department. They included the social centres for the elderly, multi-services centres, home-help services, day-care centres, and various types of homes for the elderly noted above. Other services, such as health and housing, were not as evident.

A central committee was not set up for a further five years, until April 1987, when the then LEGCO (Legislative and Executive Councils Office) Standing Panel on Welfare Services finally approved it. The central committee, with its members appointed by the secretary for health and welfare, then functioned as an advisory panel on health and social welfare services with a special focus on older people. This committee served for a year and produced the *Report of the Central Committee on Services for the Elderly* in September 1988, which still very much reflected the earlier programme plans but was a bit more elaborate. The central committee report stated the problems in services coordination, resulting in the formation of an inter-professional committee. In addition, it critically reviewed services and pinpointed policy defects in a number of areas, including inadequate funding/ provision, the horizontal and vertical coordination of services, central–district operational structures and the relationships between government and non-government organizations.

In response to the central committee's review, the Social Welfare Department drafted the 1989 five-year plan review, which further acknowledged the inadequacy of services and projected the demands. The plan emphasized community care, integrated services and family as a service unit, thereby promoting services integration and community care. It also strengthened existing services, with two pilot projects for out-reach care for single or isolated elderly people. Therefore, in spite of the problems mentioned, a distinguishable effort was made at least by the Social Welfare Department's programme and review plans, indicating the government was aware of the problems faced by "the elderly".

In the early 1990s, there was a general tendency to treat the elderly population as a priority target for special needs. The 1992, 1993 and 1994 *Governor's Policy Addresses* stated that elderly people were a service priority, justifying an extra injection of funds. Cash benefits for elderly people, such as Old Age Allowance, were raised. The last British governor, Christopher Patten, set up a Commission for Elderly Services in 1994. A report was produced after six months, in September 1994, which included a number of initiatives, such as revised and improved planning ratios for services the redefinition of old age from 60 to 65, the proposal of an old age pension scheme and the establishment of an Elderly Services Division in the Health and Welfare (H&W) Branch (renamed the H&W Bureau after 1997).

However, actual reforms were slow in the few years to 1997. The new chief executive of the HKSAR, Tung Chee-hwa, appointed Tam Yiu-chung, a legislator and a member of the Executive Committee, to head the newly-formed Elderly Commission (EC) in July 1997. The EC has been operating since then and has the following objectives:

> The primary aim and objective of the EC is to assist the HKSARG, through rendering appropriate advice, in formulating effective policies and programmes to meet the challenges brought about by an ageing population. To strengthen our care for the elderly, we need to improve their quality of and zeal for life, step up the inter-generational communications and implement the Government's policy objectives of providing the elderly with a sense of security, a sense of belonging and a feeling

of health and worthiness. (Elderly Commission, Hong
Kong 2000, p. 1):

The Elderly Commission membership includes key policy-
makers from most government departments: the Hospital
Authority, the Department of Health, the Social Welfare
Department and the Housing Department. However, the EC has
no real executive power, although it holds a respected status.
Partly because the H&W Bureau serves as its secretariat and the
secretary for health and welfare is its vice chair, corresponding
policy-making has tended to be focused on issues relating to
health and social services. The EC, between 1997 and 2001,
achieved moderate results including:

- a comprehensive overview of policy and services, drawing
  evidence from commissioned studies and consultancy reports
  (see the first *Report of the Elderly Commission 1997–1999* Elderly
  Commission, Hong Kong 2000).
- some policy innovations: long-term care was addressed via an
  Enhanced Bought Places Scheme for buying private sector places;
  home care and enhanced home-care services; a care assessment
  scheme (gatekeeping); universal housing designs; elderly
  housing preferential allocations, and out-reach health services
  and specialist health care (dementia care) for older persons
- A new policy directive, healthy ageing, has been adopted which
  de-emphasizes chronological age, emphasizing health
  promotion and quality of life.

Within its limitations, the EC has consolidated what was
needed for a framework for an policy on ageing. In a subtle way,
its first report has also acknowledged the importance of
collaboration or cooperation among departments to achieve the
policy objectives for the year 2000 and beyond.

Directions for Hong Kong's policy on ageing beyond 2000

In spite of its advances, the policy frame presented in the *Report
of the Elderly Commission 1997–1999* (ibid) and the chief executive's

Policy Address 2000 (Tung 2000) still lacks a centrally directed and centrally coordinated structure. It represents at the most a policy document of the H&W Bureau, which echoes the chief executive's pledge to promote a "sense of security", "sense of belonging" and "sense of health and worthiness" among older persons. Nevertheless, the programme initiatives documented in these papers have, for the first time, set a clear direction for future policy on ageing. In essence, "ageing in place" and "a continuum of care" will be the guiding principles for all policy and services for the elderly. These two principles will be reflected in the new programme initiatives and in the chief executive's pledges for older persons:

A sense of security. Self-reliance and family responsibility will be encouraged for those who have the resources to look after their livelihood in old age. For those who cannot, the Comprehensive Social Security Assistance (CSSA) will provide a safety net. Indeed, 14.9 per cent of the total elderly population were claiming CSSA benefits in mid-2000, indicating that CSSA is known and used by many, if not all, who need it. A Mandatory Provident Fund (MPF) came into operation in January 2001, offering additional long-term retirement protection based on employers' and employees' contributions (albeit limited at 5 per cent of salaries up to HK$20,000 per month).

A sense of belonging. Policy and services aimed at promoting a sense of belonging essentially cover housing, community support and residential care. They include a priority housing allocation scheme for families willing to live with their elderly relatives; provision of accommodation for all elderly people within two years of their application; a special housing programme for elderly tenants, including sheltered housing and a rental allowance; and the encouragement of private housing developers to target provision for elderly customers.

Residential care. This includes addressing many of the shortcomings noted earlier, such as increasing the total number of subsidized places (a net increase of 5,200 places by 2008);

improving the quality of private homes through licensing requirements, ensuring all existing homes have a licence; reducing the waiting period to 17 months for admission to homes; and the establishment of a standardized care-needs assessment scheme for elderly people requiring residential care.

Community support. This includes providing home-based care to enable the "continuum of care" at home; re-engineering home-help services through open tenders, to make them more cost-effective; improving support for carers; strengthening day-care and respite services; and special provision for dementia and for people deemed at risk of suicide.

A sense of health and worthiness. This area focuses on health, an obvious concern for an ageing population. In addition to the Hong Kong Government's promise to maintain the present level of health-care services for the needy, resources have been injected into running health promotion and health maintenance programmes for the older people in the community. These include establishing 18 new health centres for the elderly and 18 community geriatric assessment teams. In line with this is the promotion of "healthy ageing" and the EC is initiating "healthy ageing programmes" for 2001–04. Indeed, "positive ageing" and "productive ageing", two well-known gerontological concepts, are identified as two components of healthy ageing. Elderly people are encouraged to lead a positive and active life by means such as being volunteers, or by improving their relationships with their children and grandchildren.

The review so far has presented a promising picture for the formulation of a coherent ageing policy for 2000 and beyond. However, a major drawback to developing a national policy on ageing in Hong Kong has not been the lack of policy initiatives, but rather the lack of a data bank on which policy can draw for evidence, the lack of policy-to-service-delivery links, and a poor implementation process. These may be explained as follows.

The lack of comprehensive data for policy-making

Modelling itself on other advanced countries, Hong Kong is fast catching up in building a structure for elderly care. However, the severe lack of data in many related areas is hindering the development of informed policy. Data needed include more refined socio-economic and health-status characteristics of adult cohorts; information on health and social services usage and outcomes; longitudinal studies to track selected patient/service groups; data on networks and levels of support; and, finally, risk indicators and registration.

Problems in policy and in service delivery

On paper, Hong Kong clearly offers a wide range of services for older persons, but these services are neither comprehensive nor integrated in their actual operation. The main problems noted in 1996 by the Hong Kong Association of Gerontology (1996), which are largely still valid, are:

A lack of vision of the role of older persons in society, and the limitations in definition of service targets. Elderly people are seen as a burden to society, with evidence of policy "moral panic". While the policy on services for older persons is "care in the community", service targets are limited to elderly people alone, and in many instances are limited to single and/or deprived elderly persons. The Elderly Commission has evidently taken note of this and is starting to promote the concept of an "ageless society", although the effect of this initiative remains to be seen.

A lack of comprehensive and operational plans. Although "community care" has been emphasized for planning services for elderly people, government departments often mention only the importance of domiciliary care and community support services, omitting the policy commitments to make community care a reality. The government therefore needs to give clear policy statements and resource commitments to show its active pursuit of better service provision for older persons, to enable them to continue living in their own communities. The government needs to do more than just try to encourage such provisions; it needs to commit resources to them. In addition, whilst the family is depicted as the key source of caring for older persons in community care, there is little evidence of concrete services to support families in fulfilling such functions. For example, what could be more obvious than a direct cash subsidy for families to take care of their elderly members in need? Furthermore, the increase in the elderly population (in percentage and numerical terms) itself warrants a substantial reallocation of resources, yet few extra resources have been devoted in anticipation of the impact of an ageing society.

The lack of integration and coordination.   Coordination and integration of service policies have rarely been seriously discussed within or between departments. This may be attributed to the nature of the Hong Kong administrative system, in which civil servants are currently only accountable to their own department heads and policy-making has not been open to public involvement. Service policies at a departmental level are often made within the confines and expertise of a particular department, and unless a department specifically requests cross-department cooperation, it will tend to remain operationally isolated from other departments. This lack of integration and coordination sometimes raises serious problems in policy-making and resource use. It has therefore always been a problem to turn good policies into good practice. There is a recognized lack of public accountability which allows department heads to be authoritarian and even evasive in their responsibilities — even more so for NGOs. An accountability structure which incorporates public (especially users') involvement could improve this situation.

Although cooperation among or coordination of services between various departments has nevertheless frequently been on the policy agenda of departments, the actual coordination of service delivery to elderly people is easier said than done. For example, currently, when an elderly person applies for a residential place at a care and attention home, the Social Welfare Department's assessment may indicate that the applicant is more suited for an infirmary place, for which the person may then be asked to apply. The assessment by the infirmary may indicate that he or she is more suited for a care and attention home. As there are no formal channels of communication between the two sections, the elderly person can be shunted around and may end up with no service at all. It is unlikely that problems resulting from this lack of coordination at a local level can be tackled solely by central policy. What is required is for service departments to be accountable at local district levels, where services are delivered and received.

Attempts to rectify policy-service misfits: long-term care initiatives

In response to the problems or misalignments between policy and services, the H&W Bureau is attempting to reduce such discrepancies, first by planning in preparation for projected demands and, secondly, by encouraging the development of new service models for inter-disciplinary and inter-departmental collaboration. The projected increase in the population aged 65 and above from 734,100 (10.7 per cent) in 1999 to 830,200 (11.2 per cent) by 2006 has posed a significant challenge for service providers and Hong Kong as a whole. The government's response has been to see spending on elderly services increase from HK$1.58 billion (US$0.2 billion) in 1997/98 to HK$2.7 billion in 2000/01. Direct expenditure on long-term care services has risen from HK$760 million (US$ 0.8 million) in 1992/93 to HK$3.5 billion in 2000, an increase of more than four and a half times. Despite this, the debate on long-term care for older people has focused on the gap between demand and supply, which requires more policy and programme initiatives to meet the needs of the increasingly ageing population. In this respect, reforms in the funding sources and structure, and initiatives to promote a continuum of care and enhanced home care, are proposed. While these reforms and measures have aroused uncertainty and criticism among the health and social service sectors, they have also started to move in an appropriate direction in long-term care for Hong Kong, which requires fundamental changes in inter-disciplinary and inter-departmental collaboration.

Long-term care in Hong Kong

Given the current and future importance of long-term care (LTC) in Hong Kong and similar societies, this section first attempts to gauge the need for long-term care. It then continues to examine whether current provisions are meeting these needs and how new initiatives have been planned for better service, before finally looking at the crucial issues of financing.

The need for long-term care

Long-term care is generally defined, as in Chapter 1, as care delivered to individuals who are dependent on others for assistance with the basic tasks necessary for physical, mental and social functioning over a sustained period of time (Kane and Kane 2000; Phillips 2000*a*). Long-term care in Hong Kong likewise refers to the range of services usually comprising health, personal care, and social services provided to individuals who have lost the capacity to care fully for themselves and need to depend on others for a continuing period. Despite the popular tendency to equate long-term care solely with residential or institutional care, the growing recognition of the importance of community-based services, home care and respite care in providing the needed support and care has altered the current provision and long-term policy development of services for the elderly (Phillips 2000*a*).

Factors that affect the need for long-term care

The need for long-term care for elderly people in Hong Kong arises not merely as a result of the growing elderly population, but also reflects the interplay of multiple factors that affect the supply and demand for LTC in the long run (Leung 2000; Phillips 2000*b*). These include interlinked epidemiological and society-based factors.

Epidemiological transition: demographic ageing and some physical deterioration

Hong Kong currently has an elderly population of over one million aged 60 and over, which grew by 39 per cent between 1986 and 1996. It is estimated that by 2006 there will be a further increase of 23 per cent over 1996, and that by 2011 the ratio of the oldest-old (people aged 80 and over) in the local population will increase significantly. Male life expectancy in 2001 was around 77 years, and that of females almost 83 years; this is likely to increase to over 78.1 and 83.4 by 2016. A greater proportion of very elderly people and higher life expectancy generally imply heavier demands on health and social services.

It is important to note that, as discussed in Chapter 1, aggregate need for LTC is influenced not only by the ageing of the population but even more importantly by the health status of older persons, and also social conditions, including service provision. In Hong Kong, over half of the older population (aged 65 and over) have various degrees of disability and 24 per cent have mild to severe grade mental illness (Table 2.5). The rapid ageing of the society and the increase in proportion of those suffering from chronic illnesses (Table 2.6 and Table 2.7) have exerted substantial pressure on the demand for various types of LTC.

TABLE 2.5
Hong Kong: Health Problems of the Elderly Population

Health problem	Percentage of Population Aged 65+
Mental illness	24%
Physically handicapped	53%
Visual problems	64%
Hearing problems	25%

Source: Social Welfare Department, Hong Kong (11 Jabuary 2000).

TABLE 2.6
Hong Kong: Distribution of Chronic Diseases by Age and Sex (percentages)

Diagnosis	<18 Male	<18 Female	18–39 Male	18–39 Female	40–64 Male	40–64 Female	65+ Male	65+ Female
Back pain	0.4	0	0.4	1.4	9.5	13.0	24.9	34.5
Hypertension	0	0	0.4	0.6	7.2	12.4	17.8	26.9
Rheumatism	0.2	0.2	1.3	2.2	6.9	7.8	7.5	14.1
Diabetes	0	0	0	0.2	2.2	4.9	6.1	12.0
Skin problems	0.8	0.4	0.8	1.2	1.9	1.5	2.8	2.4
Peptic ulcer	0	0.4	1.1	0.7	2.0	1.6	1.9	0.8
Headache	0	0.7	0.5	1.2	1.4	2.4	1.4	1.6
Asthma	1.4	1.6	0.7	0.4	0.5	1.3	4.2	0.8
Chronic bronchitis	0.4	0.2	0.2	0.7	0.3	1.8	3.8	2.4
Heart disease	0	0	0.1	0.1	0.8	1.8	3.8	5.6
Cataract	0	0	0	0	0.3	1.0	3.8	1.6
Psychiatric illness	0	0	0.1	0.5	0.6	1.1	0	0
Stroke	0	0	0	0	0.3	0	3.8	1.6
Deafness	0	0	0	0	0.2	0.3	3.3	1.6
Thyroid disease	0	0.2	0.1	0.9	0	0.8	0.5	0

Source: Leung and Lo (1997).

TABLE 2.7
Hong Kong: Prevalence of Common Illnesses Among the Older Population

Illness	Number	Percentage
Rheumatism	504	34.2
Hypertension	474	32.2
Fracture	205	17.1
Peptic ulcer	198	13.5
Diabetes mellitus	158	10.7
Chronic bronchitis	120	8.2
Coronary heart disease	100	6.8
Hyperthyroidism	89	6.1
Urinary incontinence	72	4.9
Stroke	55	3.8
Faecal incontinence	43	2.9
Hyperparathyroidism	21	1.4

Source: Leung and Lo (1997).

Increases in dementia, depression and elderly suicide
The increase in the ageing population and longevity inevitably appear to bring an increase in age-related ailments. Mental conditions such as cognitive impairments and depression have been increasing, though they had passed largely unnoticed until recent years. Older persons with such conditions were tolerated and inadequately cared for at home or in institutions. With increased awareness of the need to treat age-related ailments, there is a rising demand for public services for conditions for which it was once thought shameful to ask for help outside the family. These include dementia, depression and suicidal tendencies. On top of physical ailments, other conditions can bring multiple problems, including behavioral or personality changes and inter-personal conflicts. For all these to be treated properly, many services have to be provided in LTC settings.

There are not reliable national figures on the prevalence of dementia. The nearest to a representative prevalence study was made in 1993 by Liu et al., using an elderly sample (over 2000 people aged 60 and above) drawn from general households. This may be supplemented by various other community-based and residential home studies conducted over recent years. Results consistently show that, among those aged 65 or above, the prevalence of moderate to severe dementia is around 4 per cent, similar to that in many other advanced countries (4–5 per cent in the general population). The estimates for prevalence in care and attention homes and in nursing homes (which provide a higher level of care) are around 37 per cent and 94 per cent respectively. It may be projected, based on a 4 per cent prevalence, that by 2016 there will be at least 43,600 elderly people with dementia (assuming a projected population of 1.09 million people aged 65 and over).

Depression is the most common psychological symptom among the elderly population, with a prevalence ranging from 5 per cent to 15 per cent estimated by various diagnostic criteria and for different cohorts. Older persons living in the community in Hong Kong have been found to have an even higher rate, ranging from 15 per cent (Chi and Boey 1994) to 70 per cent (Ngan et al. 1996); and some studies have indicated that the average is around 45 per cent (Chan 1997). In other words, almost one in two elderly people may suffer from some degree of depression in Hong Kong.

About two-thirds of those who committed suicide are thought to have had episodes of depression before they killed themselves. It seems logical then that with a high depression rate will come higher suicide rates. Hong Kong already has a high elderly suicide rate of 28 per 100,000 (as opposed to 12 in the general population), higher than that of most advanced countries (USA 20, Australia 16, New Zealand 12) but lower than Singapore (50) and rural Beijing (38) (Chi et al. 1997; Ruzicka 1998; Phillips 2000b). Not only does suicide indicate personal unhappiness and brings great pain to the people around those who die, but it also creates a series of problems and ethical concerns for those involved with the families and the deceased.

Social issues influencing the need for LTC
Apart from the challenge posed by the demographic and epidemiological changes which put pressure on long-term care provision, many social-economic changes experienced by Hong Kong during the last two decades have also probably weakened the ability of the family to take care of its elderly members. These may have therefore increased the potential need for formal, non-family based LTC. The number of nuclear families was increasing while a number of elderly people live alone (Table 2.8 and Table 2.9). There is a trend for more family members, especially women in the family, to be in employment, which has left many older people to care for themselves (Chi 1994). The reliance on a spouse as principal carer is also more problematic as people grow older, and many of course become widowed or remain single. Given that many elderly people in Hong Kong rely on social security payments because of poverty (Table 2.10), they cannot purchase domestic help like many middle-class Hong Kong citizens. When elderly people's financial ability is low yet they have to take care of themselves, they may be forced to rely on public services. This implies that the demand for LTC community supportive services or institutional care will incrementally rise once physical or cognitive abilities of the elderly population start to impair their basic self-care abilities.

TABLE 2.8
Hong Kong: Living Arrangements of the Population Aged 60 and Above, 2001

Living Arrangement	Percentage
Living alone	11.4
Living with spouse and/or children only	78.5
Living with other persons	10.0

Source: Census and Statistics Department (2002*a*).

TABLE 2.9
Hong Kong: Marital Status of Persons Aged 65 or Above, 1994

Marital Status	Male		Female		Total	
Never married	16,665	(5.0%)	17,021	(4.4%)	33,686	(4.7%)
Married	271,308	(81.7%)	191,806	(49.9%)	463,114	(64.6%)
Widowed	39,382	(11.9%)	170,243	(44.2%)	209,625	(29.2%)
Divorced/ separated	4,786	(1.4%)	5,690	(1.5%)	10,476	(1.5%)
Total	332,141	(100%)	384,760	(100%)	716,901	(100%)

Source: Hong Kong Government (1994).

TABLE 2.10
Hong Kong: Single Households Living in Poverty or Abject Poverty

Age	Abject Poverty		Poverty		Total	
0–19	—	(0%)	1,000	(0.9%)	1,000	(0.8%)
20–39	1,000	(6.3%)	46000	(40%)	47,000	(35.9%)
40–59	1,000	(6.3%)	33000	(28.7%)	34,000	(26.%)
60 & up	14,000	(87.5%)	35000	(30.4%)	48,000	(36.6%)
Total	16,000	(100%)	115,000	(100%)	131,000	(100%)

Source: Hong Kong Council of Social Services/Oxfam (1996).

However, it is wrong to assume that no family care is available for older persons in Hong Kong. In fact, many elderly people still live with their children (about 70 per cent) and, when asked, children are generally willing to take responsibility for their fair share of care. However, "fair share" is the key issue, and the disproportional lack of family support has come from the combined effects of two major processes. The pull for using public services has been evident in the increasingly high-quality services found in the public sector. Most services are provided free or at low cost. For example, for free, an elderly person can enjoy a space of 120 square feet in a care centre and receive round-the-clock attention. At home, space is at a premium and the same person may have to make do with merely 50 square feet, and would not be looked after during the day when the family goes to work. The push for the family to utilize public care has been twofold. It is expensive for an average income family to take care of an elderly person properly at home: more hours in care, fewer hours to work, hence more money spent in care and less money to bring home. It is also tiring to care for an elderly person over a long period of time at home, and this can lead to fatigue, frustration, and feelings of incapability and isolation. The typical family-caring process in Hong Kong starts with everyone in the family rushing to provide some care when the need initially arises. Then the woman (usually, the daughter or the daughter-in-law) persists for a bit longer. Finally, the family, except for the elderly person, seeks a place in a government-maintained home. Only recently has support been considered for people who take care of elderly people at home. Previously, family carers were thought of as requiring no more support than that from centre-based community services provided by the SWD.

The current system of long term-care in Hong Kong

As in most Western countries, long-term care in Hong Kong generally developed along two main streams: residential care and home/community-based care. Under the initiatives for "ageing in place" and "community care", older persons in Hong Kong are encouraged to live in their homes for as long as possible, assisted by community support services when needed. However, programme reviews commissioned by the government in recent years have revealed that the current modes and delivery of community support services have not matched the needs of families or elderly members. Worse still perhaps is the fact that about one-third of people now residing in residential homes should be able to live independently at home (Deloitte and Touche 1997). The provision of effective community LTC support services has the obvious potential to reduce the demand for LTC residential care. In this regard, government-funded LTC services are currently being re-engineered.

Residential care

Residential care can be classified according to the nature and level of care it provides — ranging from self-care hostels, aged homes, care and attention homes, nursing homes and infirmaries, which provide the highest level of care — as summarized in Table 2.11.

The wide range of caring institutions perhaps reflects the historical practice of fixing a level of care for each type of home without acknowledging the possibility of deterioration of its residents. Residents, instead of "ageing in place", are ageing in many places, sometimes sequentially as they are moved from one type of home to another. To redress the balance, the SWD has now introduced a mixed funding model, offering higher resources to operators if they care for elderly people with higher dependency. There are also support measures for retaining elderly residents whose health status is deteriorating, including a dementia supplement and infirmary care supplement (annually US$5,200 per head) for residential care homes to employ additional staff to provide better care for demented or infirm residents. There are also emergency and respite payments to provide urgent and temporary accommodation to prevent older persons from being at risk, or to offer temporary relief to their main caregivers.

The increase in the number of private homes for the aged is another significant local development. As recently as 1981, there were as few as 7 private homes for the aged, which increased to 73 in 1986 and dramatically to 256 in 1990. In 2000–01 there were

TABLE 2.11

Hong Kong: Types of Residential Care Available, 2001

Level of Care	Types of Residential Care	Service Description
L O W E S T	Elderly hostel	Provides communal living accommodation, organized programmes and round-the-clock support to older persons who are capable of self-care.
	Aged home	Provides residential care, meals and limited assistance in activities of daily living for older persons who are capable of personal or nursing care but unable to live independently in the community.
	Care and Attention home	Provides residential care, meals, personal care and limited nursing care and assistance in activities of daily living for elderly people who suffer from poor health or disabilities.
H I G H E S T	Nursing home	Provides accommodation, regular and basic medical, nursing and rehabilitative services, social support and personal care to elderly people who suffer from poor health or physical/mental disabilities.
	Infirmary	Provides medical/hospital care to elderly people who suffer from physical/mental disabilities.

Source: Social Welfare Department Hong Kong (May 2001).

over 500 private homes for the aged housing about 25,000 elderly residents — over half of the total residential care population. About 80 per cent of residents are using social security payments to pay or part-pay their charges, and the private sector will be the key provider for residential placements in the foreseeable future. The sector is willing and ready to meet the shortfall, responding to market demand, as opposed to the cumbersome government bureaucratic procedure for developing purpose-built nursing homes (it takes at least five years to build a 200-place public home). In a weak economic climate, the private sector seizes new opportunities and in a relatively short time can help to speed up the supply and eventually reduce the number of elderly people on the waiting list. Nonetheless, if opportunistic entrepreneurs are involved, the control of quality in these homes is obviously a major concern that calls for regulation, inspection and appropriate quality standards.

The sharp increase in the number of private homes for the aged may reflect the multiple effects of social, political and demographic changes during the past two decades, as initially pointed by Phillips (1988b). Public outcries for the regulation of private homes as a result of scandals are not uncommon in Hong Kong, as elsewhere, and led to the introduction of the Residential Care Homes (Elderly Persons) Ordinance, enacted in 1995. All residential care homes for the elderly must be licensed or granted a Certificate of Exemption to legitimize their operations. The Government has also tried to fill the shortfall in the public provision of residential care by buying places from qualified private homes. Table 2.12 shows the provision in 2000 of residential care in Hong Kong.

TABLE 2.12
Hong Kong: Provision of Residential Care, 2000

Types of Residential Care	Government Subvented		Self-financing		Private Profit-making	
	Units	Places	Units	Places	Units	Places
Elderly hostels	21	896		42		
Aged homes	33	7,098	42	1,393	500	25,000
Care and attention homes	72	8,992		1,594	(3,348 places	
Nursing homes	6	1,400			bought by	
Infirmary	19	1,433			government)	
Total		19,819		3,029		

Source: Social Welfare Department, Hong Kong (29 February 2000); Hong Kong Hospital Authority (2000).

The shortfall between demand and supply

With the growing need for LTC provision, a gap has grown between demand and supply (Table 2.13). In March 2002, there were some 29,000 applicants for various types of residential care services on the waiting list registered under the Residential Care Services Delivery System for the Elderly Office. In part, this is because being entered on the list is at present not difficult, and any elderly person can be placed on it following a referral by a social worker. Nevertheless, there is no indication that these referrals are inappropriate, and indeed most of the elderly people on the waiting list are in poorer physical condition than residents in NGO homes. Therefore, in order to provide these people, and others such as elderly people discharged from hospital, with suitable assistance to live at home, a frequent yet accurate means of need assessment has to be devised.

TABLE 2.13
Hong Kong: Waiting Time and Waiting List for Residential Care, 2000

Types of Residential Care Homes	Waiting Time (months)	Waiting List	
		Number	%
Elderly hostels	11	73	0.3
Aged homes	20	5,647	19.7
Care and attention homes (subvented places)	34	17,370	60.8
Private aged homes Bought places scheme Enhanced bought places scheme	10		
Nursing homes	17	5,484	19.2
Total		28,574	100.0

Source: Social Welfare Department, Hong Kong (31 March 2002).

Need assessment

Adequate provision of services requires an accurate and meaningful assessment of both existing and projected needs. It is therefore crucial for the government to adopt an assessment scheme that takes into consideration all the relevant dimensions of the client group for which services are provided. In the case of LTC, the need for such care tends to hinge on two main dimensions: the degree of the older person's physical and cognitive impairment, and the availability of informal care for him/her (Deloitte and Touche 1997). However while these may be yardsticks to distinguish between demand and need, the needs of older persons often change during the ageing process. It is hence essential to develop a comprehensive long-term plan to cater for the changing needs of the elderly population. The elderly health centres, the community geriatric and psycho-geriatric assessment schemes, and the gatekeeping (need assessment) mechanism recently developed are geared precisely to this end.

Home and community-based care

These are non-residential care and services provided for older people to enable them to continue living in their own homes or in the community for as long as possible. Despite the official emphasis on family care and community care as the core theme and policy direction of services for the elderly, the provision of services in this respect is often discrete and lacks overall strategic planning (Table 2.14).

TABLE 2.14
Provision of Community-based Services, June 2000

Types of Community-based Service	Provision (number)	Service Description
Community geriatric assessment teams	9	Act as gatekeeper to residential services — conduct pre-admission assessments of infirmary applicants and some care and attention applicants on the central waiting list.
Community nursing services	14 centres (250 nurses)	Provide nursing care and treatment for patients in their own homes.

TABLE 2.14 (continued)

Types of Community-based Service	Provision (number)	Service Description
Day-care centres	33	Provide personal care and limited nursing care to frail elderly persons living in the community during the daytime.
Home-help teams	138	On a district basis — to assist elderly with daily routines such as personal care, shopping, meal, escorts and household management. Home care teams also provide nursing care.
Home care teams	25	
Meal service teams	25	
Carers' support centers	2	Provide support, skill-training, information and recreational activities to carers, and loan of rehabilitation-aid equipment.
Day-care centres for demented older persons	4 centres, each offering 20 places	Provide day-care service and training to older clients suffering from mild to moderate senile dementia, and supportive services to carers.
Day respite service	12 centres, each, offering 3 places	Provide temporary day-care services for demented or frail older persons to provide respite relief to carers.

Source: Social Welfare Department, Hong Kong (June 2000).

Innovations in LTC

In view of the policy directives from the Hong Kong SAR Government on services for the elderly and the growing public demand for better quality and quantity in service provision, the Social Welfare Department has put into effect a number of innovative measures and programmes. These include the setting up of an enhanced home-care programme, the implementation of standardized care, a need assessment mechanism for elderly services, and a pilot project on the continuum of care in residential homes.

The Enhanced Home-care Programme
This programme initiative was introduced in 1999 by contracting out home care and meal services to bidders who could be NGO's or private profit-making companies. The emphasis is on providing good quality home care, nursing care and meals services to elderly persons living at home or in the community. It is hoped that through this new mode of contracting for services, better quality care services will be provided which should greatly reduce the future need for institutional care. The initiative is targeted at elderly people with only a moderate level of impairment, who will receive support via home helps, personal care, nursing and allied health services, along with their caregivers. By March 2000, a total of 18 service contracts valued at HK$63 million per year (US$8.5 million) for three years had been awarded to 14 non-governmental organizations.

Standardized Care Need Assessment Mechanism for elderly services
As a measure to ensure that clients' needs are matched by services and to strengthen the gate-keeping role of the social welfare professionals, a "standardized care need assessment mechanism for elderly services" has been implemented by phases since November 2000. Under this mechanism, an international standardized assessment tool (MDS-HC) is used to determine the care need of elderly people and to match them with the appropriate services.

The scope of services under this assessment mechanism includes homes for the aged , care and attention homes, nursing homes, day-care centers and home-help/home care services. All assessors are required to undertake training programmes before they are accredited to conduct assessment. Five multi-disciplinary "standardized care need assessment management offices (elderly services)" have been set up to monitor the operations of the mechanism and to handle appeals.

Pilot project on continuum of care
The objective of this pilot project is to enable residential care homes to have the flexibility of using resources to employ staff, hire services and organize therapeutic and training programmes

to cater for the changing needs of their elderly inmates. Three residential care homes for the elderly have been chosen to join the pilot project ,which will last for three years from August 2000 to July 2003.

Funding for long-term care

Modes of funding

In parallel with the consideration of policy and programmes for LTC is the crucial issue of finance. Unlike short-term or emergency care, neither the state nor the family, including the older person, can generally foot all the bills. Advanced countries with better planning talk about three or four "pillars" of finance for LTC (Phua 2000), generally identified as private savings, private insurance or pensions, public insurance or pensions and a minimum safety net of social security. Some even are now speculating on a fifth pillar, long-term care insurance. However, Hong Kong in its 150 years of history has not developed long-term social costs planning; it has some 20 years' minimum subsistence guaranteed through social security payments, and a fairly comprehensive but expensive health and social care system. As noted earlier, only in 2000 was a contributory Mandatory Provident Fund (MPF) retirement financing scheme introduced, which is expected to mature only after 30 or 40 years. It is an agreed economic aim in Hong Kong that direct taxation remain low, but it is not difficult to foresee the escalating expenditure on LTC pressurizing this. Hong Kong citizens have been assured that there is no immediate financial crisis in service provision, but a longer perspective and effective strategies for financing LTC must be looked at. The public were consulted on the possibility of implementing contributory savings for health services and long-term care insurance (both at 1–2 per cent of income) at the beginning of 2001, but decisions have been deferred because of the global economic downturn. It seems that in the interim, for services to remain at their present quality and quantity, expenditure will have to be carefully controlled and used efficiently and effectively. As financial subsidies create the primary pressure for changes in NGOs and executive departments, the

SAR government is reviewing present sources and methods of funding, and this may be seen as part of a wider review of fiscal policy.

Sources of funding
In Hong Kong, the cost for the provision of LTC (including formal residential and community services) for older persons is borne mainly by the government from general revenue, although charitable institutions also provide some support. Most service users contribute only a relatively small portion of the full costs of care. As noted, only recently has the possibility of introducing a social insurance/contributory scheme to pay in part towards the medical costs of the local population been considered. There is currently little or no private and social insurance available locally for LTC for older persons, and this is especially so for residential care (some people have limited shorter-term cover under private health insurance schemes).

Before 1999, government funding for elderly services was mainly via direct subventions to service providers (not users), most of which are non-governmental organizations. The government's role has thus been to act as a fund-provider to the subvented sector, and in some instances as a direct service provider. Given the changing socio-economic situation and prospects of Hong Kong, as well as growing calls for budget control and cuts in welfare expenditure, the government has started to seek alternative ways to deliver and pay for the cost of current and projected demands for long-term care for older persons. The government is now working on selected service items which, for those who can afford it, can be charged at a higher rate. By so doing, it is hoped that the current expenditure can be capped and some users may be redirected to private sectors, or may be encouraged to use services more responsibly.

Methods of funding
One of the first initiatives by the government to seek alternative ways for sponsoring LTC for older persons was the contracting out of home help and home care service in 1999, and an open bidding exercise in 2000 to run 6 nursing homes. It has been hoped that such measures will increase cost-effectiveness and

improve the quality of service, by encouraging competition among subvented and private sectors and by spurring providers to seek more efficient means of delivery. The views of a 1997 consultant study have largely been adopted; it recommended that the private sector should be encouraged into the provision of services for the elderly despite concerns over the quality of many private homes for the aged (Deloitte and Touche 1997). It is reasoned that once service provision for the elderly evolves into a competitive market, the role of the government will change to become a purchaser of services. It will be then in a stronger position to negotiate better quality of service at lower costs, whilst still retaining the stick of legislation. The NGO and private providers, on the other hand, would be forced to generate and experiment with innovative ways of service delivery to ensure they are not left out in the bidding process. It is also through such a bidding process that pricing — delineated into costs and profits — is revealed. For example, it was noted in 2000 that a meal provided by the meals-on-wheels standard home-help team costs around US$11, while an ordinary three-course lunch on the street costs half that amount or less.

Although competition has the potential to improve the quality of service, the experience of other countries that have experimented with this area of health sector reform is ambiguous. It is clear that effective monitoring and evaluation are crucial to maintain quality and to avoid scandals of labour exploitation or corruption, as occurred in Hong Kong in 2000 in the contracting out of cleaning services and home purchasing schemes. In this regard, the SWD has been pushing since 1997 for a quality assurance: service quality standards (SQS). This, together with a funding and services agreement (FSA), should help to maintain service standards whilst making sure service funding is used appropriately.

In addition to funding and contracting initiatives, the autonomy of older citizens to make choices about the type of care they want and need should also be a significant factor in funding reforms, as well as being an indicator of service quality. The suggestion that "funding goes with the older person" implies that a certain sum in direct subsidy will be given to older clients who can then choose their own combination of care provision, which would encourage better service matching. For example, in the Hong Kong context, older persons could use the subsidy to hire a domestic helper at around US$500 per month to provide personal care at home. Alternatively, they may choose to pay a family member or friend to do the job so as to reduce the financial burden on the family whilst retaining the personal touch. It may be noted that the per capita level of government subsidy in 2001–02 for subvented nursing homes was approximately US$1,700 per month, which exceeded the Hong Kong median income (US$1,200).

Adjusting direct subsidies according to an elderly person's condition might also encourage a fairer funding formula to residential homes which accommodate more frail residents. A case-mix funding mode could enable the formal funding of the mixture of cases that currently exists in most residential homes. They could thereby be converted into multi-purpose homes, allowing a true "ageing in place" for their residents.

The above initiatives in LTC funding and approaches have been carefully studied. Some have been effective in pilot tests whilst some remain under debate by service providers, policy-makers and parties interested in the welfare of older persons.

Conclusion

Today's national policy on ageing in Hong Kong represents a piecemeal evolution over thirty years. Policy over the past decade has definitely become more coherent and considered. Today, this growing coherence represents the efforts of the chief executive, the Elderly Commission (EC) and the Health and Welfare Bureau. The EC has so far developed guidelines principally for the three executive departments: the Hospital Authority (HA) for hospital treatment and rehabilitation, the Department of Health for health promotion and disease prevention, and the Social Welfare Department for personal social services. Other departments still tend to implement complementary yet essentially independent policies to improve services for older persons.

Whilst policy is undoubtedly emerging, many issues remain to be tackled in terms of the health and social needs of older persons. The Hong Kong SAR government is also going through a learning process in attempting to meet these needs through policy formulation and implementation. Policy imperatives to be addressed include the need for data for policy-making and evaluation, the poor integration within and between health and social services providers, which has resulted in a fragmented delivery of services, and the lack of clear operational or policy implementation plans for service delivery. Some policy and service initiatives are being taken to address these challenges, especially in view of the projected rapid increase in the elderly population.

An important point for policymaking and the potential transfer of initiatives from other systems is that, whilst the demographic ageing of Hong Kong's population is similar to that in many other advanced countries (Phillips 2000b), there are subtle characteristics driving a potentially heavier demand for long-term care than in some. For example, the physical status of Hong Kong's elderly population indicates a need for better care, while their psychological status is not very good, with a high incidence of depression and suicide (although the prevalence of dementia is roughly comparable with other countries). The socio-economic status of the current elderly cohorts is also not strong. The majority of today's older persons in Hong Kong are relatively poor without access to a decent pension; given limited state financial support, they can be regarded as an "interim generation" (Phillips 2000b). This is more so as families' ability to help is becoming more limited; most children cannot look after their elderly parents for financial and other reasons; such as the small size of housing units. The overall effect is a heavy demand for long-term care paid for by the state.

The Hong Kong SAR Government has tried to base the development of LTC care on the principle of "ageing in place" — that is, elderly people should live with their families or in a familiar environment for as long as possible. This principle has been effectively underpinned Hong Kong's social welfare policy since 1977, reasserted in the 1991 White Paper and in many policy statements since then. Whilst Chinese tradition also assumes the readiness of the family to care, the fact that more families unable or unwilling to do so, coupled with many more older persons themselves asking for residential care, has made the grave shortage in home places become evident. The government has responded to such needs by building different types of residential homes. However, recent reviews on LTC provision indicate that there is a need to encourage realistic community care and support, and to revamp residential care. A greater emphasis is being put on the role of community support services in maintaining older persons in the community. At the same time, residential care types are increasingly considered in terms of matching residents' levels of dependency, resulting in the emergence of a more refined system of need assessment and integrated service delivery.

To deal with the policy and practical changes and the challenges ahead, the Hong Kong Government has considered, under the need to cap expenditure, new sources and methods of financing long-term care. The new mode suggested can be described as a "mixed economy of provision" — services for older persons will be delivered by a mixture of public, private and voluntary providers, with increased charges for selected items or selected user groups. In order to maintain the present level of service quality and quantity, methods of funding the services are linked with a quality assurance process, user choices and reasonable pricing. It is clear, therefore, that while policy initiatives on ageing have been evident in the past few years, their effects remain to be seen.

3

National Policies on Ageing in Korea

Sung-Jae Choi

Introduction

Social policies are usually formulated and developed as measures to solve or prevent social problems. It was at the turn of the 1970s that a set of features associated with ageing began to be perceived as a social problem in Korea. Over the past thirty years since the problem — or challenge — of ageing become perceived as a social issue, there seem to have existed some important factors that have contributed to population ageing as being defined as serious social problem.

The increase in the sheer number and proportion of elderly Koreans has been conspicuous, and twenty-five years into the first of the current century, the increase is expected to be unprecedented. Gigantic social changes, including institutional and structural rearrangements, which have taken place alongside the rapid modernization of Korea over the past thirty years, could not be countered by individuals or families. Families, which have generally been the safety net for older persons, are now challenged, threatened, assaulted and eroded in terms of both structure and function. Social and familial values of filial piety, familism and communalism are apparently withering away, and individualism and an orientation towards the nuclear family are developing and expanding in their place.

Ageing is quite widely regarded as a problem in Korea, one caused by societal factors rather than individual or familial factors. This becoming serious, and it shows in many different ways. A variety of social policies for older persons and their families are needed to tackle the problem. This chapter examines population ageing and provides an overview of national policies on ageing, particularly long-term care needs and policies, in Korea.

Population ageing in Korea

Changes in fertility and mortality rates in a given society are associated with the process of demographic transition often accompanying the change from an agrarian to an industrialized-urbanized state (Kim 1996). Modernization is often said to bring about further demographic transition, facilitated by a reduction in both fertility and mortality rates. Since the early 1960s, when Korean society began to modernize rapidly with the launch of a five-year economic development plan and family planning as a national policy, fertility and mortality in Korea have continually declined. Alongside the decline of fertility and mortality, Koreans' life expectancy at birth has substantially increased and consequently the sheer number and proportion of older persons has greatly increased over the past 40 years. As shown in Table 3.1, life expectancy at birth for men and women increased from 51.1 years and 53.7 years in 1960, to 72.1 and 79.5 years respectively in 2000.

TABLE 3.1
Korea: Actual and Estimated Life Expectancy at Birth, 1960–2020

Year	Mean	Male	Female
1960	52.4	51.1	53.7
1970	63.2	59.8	66.7
1980	65.8	62.7	69.9
1990	71.7	67.7	75.9
1995	73.5	69.6	77.4
2000	75.9	72.1	79.5
2010	78.8	75.5	82.2
2020	80.7	77.5	84.1
2030	81.5	78.4	84.8

Source: National Statistical Office, Korea (2000).

These figures are expected to reach 78.4 and 84.8 years respectively in 2030.

Alongside the lengthening of life expectancy, the proportion of older persons in the population aged 65 and over has also greatly increased, from 2.9 per cent in 1960 to 7.2 per cent in 2000. This percentage is projected to reach 10.7 per cent in 2010, 15.1 per cent in 2020 and 23.1 per cent in 2030 (Table 3.2). It is also estimated that it would take only 19 years for the proportion of the population aged 65 and over to increase from 7 per cent to 14 per cent. By contrast, this took 85 years to achieve in Sweden and 24 years in Japan (National Statistical Office, Korea 2001). This rate of population ageing in Korea is thus much faster compared to that of many other countries, and implies that the rapidity of population ageing will be greatly accelerated in the first quarter of the twenty-first century.

Looking at the population aged 65 and over, the higher the age bracket the faster the rate of increase (Table 3.2). This means

TABLE 3.2
Korea: Actual and Estimated Numbers and Proportions of Elderly Population, 1960–2030

	Elderly Population (A) (in thousands)				Elderly Population Ratio (A/Total Population)				Rate of Increase of the Elderly Population, past 5 years			
Year	65+	70+	75+	80+	65+	70+	75+	80+	65+	70+	75+	80+
1960	726	381	170	59	2.9	1.5	0.7	0.2	—	—	—	—
1965	881	477	232	80	3.1	1.7	0.8	0.3	21.3	25.2	36.5	35.6
1970	991	563	251	101	3.1	1.7	0.8	0.3	12.5	18.0	8.2	26.2
1975	1,217	679	344	139	3.4	1.9	1.0	0.4	22.8	20.6	44.6	37.6
1980	1,456	832	406	178	3.8	2.2	1.1	0.5	19.6	22.5	22.5	28.0
1985	1,742	1,030	523	215	4.3	2.5	1.3	0.5	19.6	23.8	28.8	20.8
1990	2,195	1,294	695	302	5.1	3.0	1.6	0.7	26.0	25.6	32.9	40.5
1995	2,657	1,608	842	382	5.9	3.8	1.9	0.8	21.0	24.3	21.2	26.5
2000	3,395	2,014	1,091	483	7.2	4.3	2.3	1.0	26.9	25.2	29.6	26.4
2005	4,366	2,667	1,445	686	9.0	5.5	3.0	1.4	28.6	32.4	32.4	42.0
2010	5,302	3,514	1,996	957	10.7	7.1	4.0	1.9	21.4	31.8	38.1	38.8
2015	6,345	4,262	2,642	1,352	12.6	8.5	5.3	2.7	19.7	21.3	32.4	39.5
2020	7,667	5,100	3,195	1,804	15.1	10.1	6.3	3.6	20.8	19.7	20.9	41.3
2025	9,689	6,177	3,812	2,156	19.1	12.2	7.5	4.3	26.4	21.1	19.4	19.5
2030	11,604	7,892	4,646	2,571	23.1	15.7	9.2	5.1	19.8	28.8	21.9	19.2

Source: National Statistical Office, Korea (2001).

that the oldest-old are the fastest growing segment among the elderly population. According to a national survey, in 1998, Koreans' life expectancy was 74.4 years, although their active life expectancy was only 64.3 years (Ministry of Health and Welfare Korea 2000*b*). This means that Koreans tend to live with diseases and/or disabilities for the last ten years of their life. Koreans' dependent life expectancy is likely to be further extended as their life expectancy is extended, and the disabled portion of their life expectancy may increase faster than the healthy and active portion.

Health status of elderly Koreans

As people age, in general, active life expectancy increases but dependent life expectancy also increases. Hence, the dependent period in the later part of old age is becoming a universal and normal life cycle (Elder et al. 1996; OECD 1997). Not only do older persons living a dependent life require health care, but many may also need social care to assist their daily living. As elderly people's age advances, their level of activities of daily living (ADL) including dressing, bathing, toileting, etc. and instrumental activities of daily living (IADL) including shopping, preparing food, house-keeping, doing laundry, etc., tends to decrease, as is shown in Figure 3.1 (Chung et al. 1998).

It is usually people with limitations in ADL that need care, particularly long-term care (LTC). Among the total elderly population of Koreans aged 65 and over, those who have limitations in ADL (F in Figure 3.1) are estimated to be about 32 per cent. Approximately 25 per cent of people aged 65–69, 32 per cent aged 70–74 and 41 per cent aged 75 have problems in their ADL. Some 3.5 per cent of all elderly Koreans aged 65 and over are estimated to be bedridden (H in Figure 3.1). If looked at by age group, it may be seen that about 2 per cent of people aged 65–69, 4.6 per cent of those aged 70–74 and 4.4 per cent aged 75 and over are bedridden. Persons with limitations only in IADL, not in ADL (E in Figure 3.1) among the total elderly Korean population are estimated to be 11.5 per cent. This ranges considerably from 4.3 per cent of those aged 65–69, 11 per cent of those aged 70–74 and 22 per cent aged 75 with limitations in IADL.

FIGURE 3.1
Korea: Physical Health Status of Older Persons

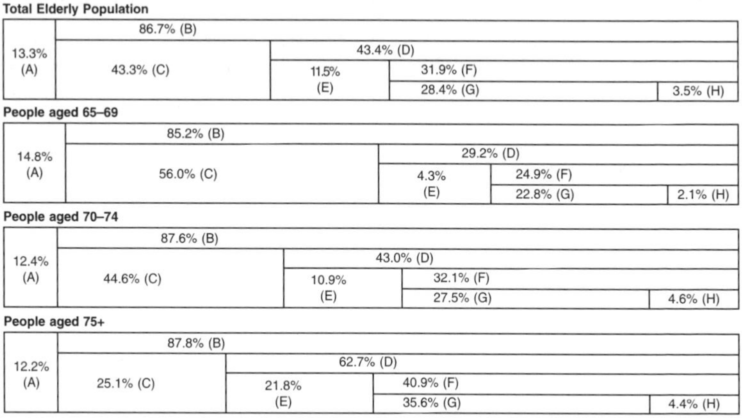

Total Elderly Population

	86.7% (B)				
13.3% (A)	43.3% (C)		43.4% (D)		
		11.5% (E)	31.9% (F)		
			28.4% (G)		3.5% (H)

People aged 65–69

	85.2% (B)				
14.8% (A)	56.0% (C)		29.2% (D)		
		4.3% (E)	24.9% (F)		
			22.8% (G)		2.1% (H)

People aged 70–74

	87.6% (B)				
12.4% (A)	44.6% (C)		43.0% (D)		
		10.9% (E)	32.1% (F)		
			27.5% (G)		4.6% (H)

People aged 75+

	87.8% (B)				
12.2% (A)	25.1% (C)		62.7% (D)		
		21.8% (E)	40.9% (F)		
			35.6% (G)		4.4% (H)

Key:
A: Healthy and living independently
B: Having chronic illness
C: Having chronic illness but living independently
H: Limitations in all (6) activities of ADL
D: Limitations in IADL
E: Limitation only in IADL
F: Limitations only in ADL
G: Limitation in 1–5 activities of ADL

Source: Chung et al. (1998).

As people get older, they may become not only physically impaired but also mentally impaired. In particular, the prevalence of senile dementia is apparently increasing with demographic ageing in Korea (Table 3.3). The proportion of elderly Koreans with dementia was estimated to be 8.2 per cent of older persons aged 65 and over in 2000, and is projected rise to 8.6 per cent in 2010 and 9.0 per cent in 2020 (Byun et al. 1997).

TABLE 3.3
Korea: Prevalence Rate of Senile Dementia among Elderly Koreans

Studies	Total	65–69	70–74	75–79	80+
Park and Koh	11.3	3.1	7.0	16.2	38.9
Seoul National University	9.5	3.7	6.7	14.9	27.2
Bae	7.0	5.2	12.2	17.0	35.2

Sources: Park and Koh (1991); Seoul National University (1995); Bae (1999).

It is not only people with physical impairments, but also often those with mental impairments who will need care, particularly long-term care. As noted in Chapter 1, almost everywhere, LTC is provided by both informal and/or formal care systems. Currently, in Korea, the majority of care is informal; almost all elderly Koreans are cared for mainly by families, relatives, neighbours and others, in various circumstances. What seems certain is that the proportion of those who utilize formal care services will inevitably increase. However, the numbers cared for by the informal care system will continue to outnumber those utilizing formal care services in the foreseeable future. In estimating the formal care needs of older persons, the existence and extent of informal care systems and dependency levels of older persons are regarded as the most crucial factors (Ministry of Health and Welfare Korea 2000b). In addition, LTC needs of older persons are also influenced by people's degree of mental as well as physical impairment.

A recent study conducted by the LTC Policy Planning Committee, Ministry of Health and Welfare (2000), estimated the proportion and number of older persons needing formal long-term care. Because no reliable statistical data exist to estimate the proportion of mentally impaired elderly people in Korea, the study estimated long-term care needs only in terms of physical health, from survey research conducted on a national sample of 2,535 Koreans aged 65 and over in 1998. The estimated proportion and number of those who needed long-term care is shown in Table 3.4 and Table 3.5. Dependency was measured by the level of IADL and ADL. A low dependency level indicates problems in only IADL; a medium dependency level indicates problems in one to five out of six items of behaviour (bathing, dressing, having meals;) and soon and a high dependency level indicates problems in all six behaviours.

In 1998, 19 per cent of elderly Koreans were estimated to be in potential need of LTC. This proportion may increase as the lifespan and the sheer number of elderly Koreans increases. If the proportion of mentally impaired elderly people who are not physically impaired are also included, the proportion and the number in need of care would have increased by some extent.

TABLE 3.4
Korea: Estimated Proportions of Older Persons Who Need Long-term Care

Level of dependency	Older Persons in the Community						Older Persons in Institutions	Total
	Living alone without carers	Living with carers						
		Spouse carers		Adult child carers				
		Aged 70 and over	Aged Under 70	Both adult child and spouse working	Only adult child working	Sub-total		
Low	0.4	0.6	0.8	2.8	2.6	7.3	19.1	7.2
Medium	2.0	1.0	1.7	2.9	2.6	10.1	40.1	10.3
High	1.5	0.3	0.2	0.5	0.4	1.5	1.5	1.5
Total	2.5	1.9	2.7	6.2	5.6	18.9	60.7	19.0

Source: LTC Policy Planning Committee, Ministry of Health and Welfare, Korea (2000).

TABLE 3.5
Korea: Estimated Numbers of Older Persons Who Need Long-term Care

Level of dependency	Older Persons in the Community						Older Persons in Institutions	Total
	Living alone without carers	Living with carers						
		Spouse carers		Adult child carers				
		Aged 70 and over	Aged Under 70	Both adult child and spouse working	Only adult child working	Sub-total		
Low	13,442	20,163	26,884	94,725	86,740	241,954	1,931	243,885
Medium	67,209	33,065	57,128	96,479	88,346	342,762	4,055	346,822
High	3,360	10,018	6,721	15,787	14,457	50,407	152	50,559
Total	84,011	63,849	90,732	206,991	189,543	635,126	6,138	641,259

Source: LTC Policy Planning Committee, Ministry of Health and Welfare, Korea (2000).

Indeed, a study of older persons in the community receiving LTC services revealed that about 12 per cent of the respondents were people who did not have physical impairments but only mental impairment (Rhee 1999).

Development of policy for older persons in Korea

The historical development of social policies for older persons in Korea can be divided into five main stages: prior to the 1960s, the 1960s, the 1970s, the 1980s, and the 1990s and after.

Prior to the 1960s

No modern type of welfare programme for older persons was instituted until 1944, when a system of public assistance was created by the Korean Relief Order on the instructions of the Japanese colonial government. With this programme, poor elderly people living in institutions and communities could be provided with some assistance from the government. The first elderly institution was opened in 1918, and later 8 more until Japanese colonial rule came to an end in 1945 (Park 1999). During this colonial period, the most serious social problem was poverty, which could not be solved systematically due to budget constraints and the harsh treatment of Koreans by the colonial government.

The 1960s

Throughout the 1950s and 1960s, after liberation from Japanese rule in 1945, the most serious aspects associated with ageing were also related to poverty. Programmes for older persons therefore consisted only of institutional care and in-home relief based on the public assistance law. It was notable that the Retirement Benefit system for both private and public companies was instituted by the legislation of the Labour Standard Law in 1953. During the 1960s, two social insurance programmes for retirement income in old age were instituted: the Government Employees Pension (GEP) in 1960 and the Military Servicemen's

Pension (MSP) in 1963. However, these two programmes only covered a very small proportion of the total number of Korean employees.

The 1970s

At the start of the 1970s, a set of issues associated with ageing began to be recognized as social problems (Hyun 1992). During this period, the patterns of issues related to ageing were beginning to diversify into economic problems, health care problems, alienation from the family and society, role losses and use of leisure time and mandatory retirement at the comparatively early age of 55. However, not all aspects of these problems associated with ageing were given serious recognition. Institutions catering for older persons were still not specialized in any concrete way — that is, homes for the aged were not differentiated from nursing homes. In 1975, another pension programme, the Private School Teachers' Pension (PSTP) was instituted to secure the retirement incomes of this group of employees.

Since the securing of medical expenses was a foremost issue, a medical insurance programme for the general public was instituted in 1977 and another, for government employees and private school teachers, in 1979. In the same year, a medical assistance programme, which was a kind of public assistance programme for the poor, was also created. In the two medical insurance programmes, older persons could be covered as the insured or as family members of the insured.

The 1980s

Modernization triggered by economic development plans and their successful implementation are felt to have resulted in family disorganization, women's increasing participation in the labour force, deterioration of traditional family values and conflicts in caring for elderly parents. From the early 1980s, associated with these phenomena, the issues of ageing became both more diversified and more serious. Accordingly, the problem of ageing began to be more widely recognized as one of Korea's most serious social problems. In particular, care of frail and ill older persons in the home emerged as an issue, in addition to the higher medical expenses involved. Following the efforts of many elderly leaders from voluntary elderly service organizations and from the congress itself, the Elderly Welfare Law was enacted in 1981.

As the general public began to recognize ageing as a serious social problem, they became much more concerned with the issue of retirement income in old age. In response to this issue, a public old-age-pension system created by the National Pension Law was instituted in 1988. As measures to promote the employment of elderly people, the Ministry of Health and Welfare instituted the Elderly Job Bank (renamed the Elderly Employment Centres in 1997) and the Elderly Workshop programmes, which operate independently of the Elderly Welfare Law.

Until 1985, there were no official nursing homes — differentiated from homes for the aged to accommodate elderly people in relatively good health — even though the Elderly Welfare Law enacted in 1981 stipulated a requirement for both nursing homes and homes for the aged separately. Since 1986, nursing homes have begun to be differentiated from homes for the aged; however, many homes for the aged were not differentiated from nursing homes until the early 1990s. For a number of reasons, it is not easy for elderly residents of homes for the aged to transfer to nursing homes when they begin to require LTC services. Thus, a significant proportion of elderly residents of the homes for the aged still have to receive long-term care at their present institutions. It may therefore be appropriate to include homes for the aged in the definition of institutions providing long-term care in Korea.

Institutional care for the aged in Korea was limited to those with low-incomes until the end of the 1980s, because there existed no fee-charging homes. This was in spite of the fact that the Elderly Welfare Law stipulated that fee-charging homes were permitted at the time of its enactment in 1981. In 1989 and 1993, the Elderly Welfare Law was amended to stipulate institutional care services for those of the middle and upper classes who could afford to pay fees.

As problems associated with ageing became increasingly diversified and more widely recognized in this period, from the mid-1980s, community care as an alternative to institutional care also began to receive public attention. Until that time, community care had not received much consideration from either academic or service fields. Community care service in Korean society began as a form of home-help service in 1987, with the initiation of a voluntary elderly-welfare agency's provision of volunteer home helpers. From 1987 to 1992, the Korean government provided financial assistance to several elderly-welfare agencies that offered home help and adult day-care services on an experimental basis. In 1993, the Elderly Welfare Law was revised to stipulate three kinds of community care services: home help, adult day-care and short-stay care. The actual term stipulated in the law in 1993 was "in-home care", not "community care". Since the term " in-home care services" can be included in "community care", it would be more appropriate to use the term "community care" rather than "in-home care". Community care services have been limited to these three kinds until the present day.

In home care and/or community care services were needed not only for low-income people but also for middle- and upper-income elderly people. Since home-help services, which became statutory services, were limited to low-income older persons, there were no appropriate home-help services for middle-and upper-income people even though they were willing to pay for them. In relation to these paid services, considerable debate emerged on the roles of social and economic markets and the domains of both markets in providing services for older persons.

The 1990s and after

With demographic ageing and the lengthening of life spans, diseases specific to older persons emerged, many chronic and degenerative in nature. Accordingly, caring for older persons at home, particularly caring for those needing LTC, has emerged as one of the most challenging issues associated with ageing.

As demographic ageing advanced, concerns about the future depletion of national pension funds began to be voiced, because the pension system was originally designed to be a scheme of lower contributions and higher benefits. In response to these concerns, the National Pension Law was amended to reduce the benefit from a 70 per cent to a 60 per cent rate of earning replacement in the case of 40 years' contributions, and to lower the minimum required period of contributions to be eligible for any kind of old-age pension (but not for a normal old-age pension) from 20 years to 10 years. As a supplementary measure to improve the income status of older workers through re-employment, the Older Workers Employment Promotion Law was enacted and came into force in 1992.

In order to guarantee a minimum living standard, the existing public assistance law (Livelihood Protection Law) was recodified into the National Basic Livelihood Security Law (NBLS) in 1999, coming into force in October 2000. This new law purports to actually guarantee a minimum living standard to all Koreans and to recognize citizens' rights to a minimum living standard. With this new public assistance law, a minimum living standard of elderly Koreans was also to be secured.

Though the old-age-pension system (National Pension) was instituted in 1988, people who had already reached pensionable age and so could not be insured under the system could not benefit from it (the pension system is to mature in 2008 after 20 years' contributions). Immediately after the inception of the National Pension (NP) programme, the issue was raised of the inequitable treatment of those who could not be insured simply due to the fact that they were aged 60 and over at the time of the pension system's inception. To compensate for this, the Old Age Allowance (OAA) was instituted in 1991 — although due to limited budgets the OAA was to be provided to low-income elderly people only. In this sense, the OAA was a kind of public assistance, rather than a universal provision given regardless of economic conditions. In 1997, this old-age allowance changed to the Elder-Respect Pension, which intended to compensate for the inequitable treatment of current pensioners. In addition, its coverage was expanded to include not only low-income elderly people and those whose incomes were above the poverty line, but also those whose income was under 65 per cent of the average monthly income for urban workers' households.

In order to solve the financial and management problems of the two medical insurance schemes, which covered elderly people as the insured or as the family members of the insured, the two systems were integrated into one, National Health Insurance (NHI), in 2000.

Because of the prevailing mandatory retirement at the early age of 55, a majority of retired Korean workers suffer serious economic problems. A majority also express a keen desire to continue to be able to engage in work (Chung et al. 1998). In order to promote older workers' employment, the Older Workers Employment Promotion Law was enacted in 1992.

Another amendment to the Elderly Welfare Law in 1997 newly categorized welfare facilities for the elderly into four groups:

1. Housing welfare facilities
2. Health care facilities
3. Community care facilities
4. Leisure facilities.

Of these four groups, all except leisure facilities for the elderly belong to long-term care provision.

Housing welfare facilities for older persons were categorized into five subgroups:

1. Free homes for the aged
2. Low-fee-charging homes for the aged
3. Full-fee-charging homes for the aged
4. Low-fee-charging welfare housing for the elderly
5. Full-fee-charging welfare housing for the elderly.

Homes for the aged were categorized into three kinds, health care facilities for the elderly were categorized into six, and community welfare facilities were categorized into three kinds.

With the amendment of the Elderly Welfare Law, adult day-care services and short-stay services (respite services) were instituted in 1993 and have since been expanded. All three kinds of community care services (home-help, adult day-care and short-stay services) are mainly limited to low-income elderly people.

Visiting nurse services, which are stipulated in the Medical Service Law and the Community Health Law but which have not been created as community care services for older persons, started in 1994 on an experimental basis, and have been expanded to all public health centres and some general hospitals. An amendment to the Medical Service Law in 1994 instituted nursing hospitals as facilities for LTC. Nursing hospitals are designed to hospitalize those who need LTC for more than 30 days.

Since the 1990s, the Korean government has recognized the importance of home and community care services, but in fact it has not paid sufficient attention to their expansion. During the 1990s, nursing care facilities increased fivefold. This means that the demand for nursing care services has increased, although it also indicates that government policies are still focusing on institutional rather than community care. Approaching the end of the 1990s, the general public and the government became aware of the importance of long-term care services for older persons. In response to these needs, the government established a policy-planning committee for long-term care at the Ministry of Health and Welfare in 2000. The first report of the committee issued in 2000 recommended the government to set up mid-and long-term policy development plans for long-term care, and identified some important basic research projects.

Current national policies for older persons

Almost all of the national policies and programmes for the welfare of older persons are currently planned and implemented by the Ministry of Health and Welfare. Social insurance programmes for income maintenance and medical services, and social service programmes for older persons are planned by the Ministry of Health and Welfare and implemented through the Ministry of Government Administration and Home Affairs. In addition to these two government ministries, there are other ministries dealing with policies and programmes related to older persons. The Ministry of Labour deals with the employment of older workers aged between 55 and 64; the Ministry of National Defence deals with the Military Servicemen's Pension; whilst the Veterans

Administration is in charge of veterans' pensions. The Ministry of Government Administration and Home Affairs deals with government employees' pensions, and the Ministry of Education deals with the Private School Teachers Pension. Housing services for poor elderly people are dealt with by the Ministry of Construction and Transportation.

Social welfare policy measures to respond to problems associated with ageing have emerged. The four major sets of needs associated with ageing are economic issues; health care needs; role loss and leisure problems; and social-psychological alienation and conflict problems (Choi 1996). Social welfare policies for older persons can be grouped into four principal categories of concern: income maintenance, health care, housing and social services. Therefore, social welfare policies may be formulated corresponding to these four groups of problems, and the resulting programmes may be reviewed in order to see whether they adequately respond to these challenges of ageing.

The social welfare problems in each category listed above will now be examined around the four basic dimensions of policy issues: coverage and eligibility requirements, benefit provisions, financial systems and delivery systems (Gilbert and Terrell 1998).

Income maintenance programmes

Public pensions
There are four public pension programmes that are designed to operate as contributory social insurance schemes: National Pension (NP), Government Employee Pension (GEP), Military Servicemen's Pension (MSP) and the Private School Teachers Pension (PSTP). The three occupation-specific pensions (GEP, MSP and PSTP) cover only 6.2 per cent of the total number of Korean workers, and the National Pension (NP) is therefore the main old-age-pension programme covering the majority of Korean workers.

However, as noted earlier, since the NP programme only began in 1988, most older persons currently aged 60 and over cannot be beneficiaries, as the pension required 20 years of contributions until 1998 when the requirement changed to 10 years. Although the NP also covers invalidity and survivor's pensions, its main function is to provide the old-age pension. In addition to the basic requirements, to have accrued 10–20 years of contributions and to be 60 years old, there are additionally some special categories in the old-age pension which also warrant eligibility.

The NP programme is financed by contributions from the employee's wages and the employer's liability for general workers; for the self-employed, it is financed only by their contributions (they pay double the employees' share) and by the contribution from the employees' income and a flat rate of government assistance for workers in agriculture and fisheries. As of 2001, about 16 million or 76.2 per cent of Korean workers were compulsorily covered by the NP programme but only 447,000 people, or 8.6 per cent, of elderly Koreans aged 60 and over were recipients of the old-age pension.

Public assistance programme
The National Basic Livelihood Security Programme (NBLS), a cash payment scheme, is a public assistance programme designed to guarantee a minimum standard of living for all Koreans. To be eligible for the NBLS programme, an elderly person must be below the poverty line, have no one legally responsible for supporting him or her or, if the elderly person does have someone legally responsible, that person must be unable to work. The NBLS stipulates five categories of benefits for elderly people: livelihood, medical, housing, self-reliance and funeral assistance. The central government contributes 80 per cent of the programme costs, with the remaining 20 per cent being shared by local government. As of 2001, older persons aged 65 and over made up 18.0 per cent of recipients of NBLS benefits and elderly recipients of NBLS benefits were 8 per cent of all elderly Koreans aged 65 and over.

Another programme providing benefits in kind to poor elderly people is the congregate meal service. This is designed to provide lunch for poor older persons who cannot pay for their meal or who cannot have lunch at home for various reasons. In 2001, there were nationally 841 places providing lunch to 841,000 elderly Koreans.

Elder-Respect Pension

The Elder-Respect Pension (ERP) is a non-contributory pension programme financed by both the central and local governments. Eligible persons for the ERP should not be covered by any other kind of public pension, and must be 65 years old and over, have a mean household income of below 65 per cent of the mean income of individual members of urban workers' households, and have household assets below 140 per cent of the assets limit of households eligible for self-reliance assistance from the NBLS. The central government contributes 50–70 per cent of the programme costs, with the remaining 30–50 per cent shared by local government. In 2001, 715,000 elderly Koreans received benefits from the ERP.

Senior Discount Programmes

The Senior Discount Programmes provide elderly people with discounts on public transport (operated by the government) and on admission to public facilities such as parks and museums, and also provides elderly people with a quantity of cash for use as a transport allowance. This programme is the only universal provision to all elderly persons aged 65 and over that is financed entirely by local government.

Employment promotion programmes

There are five kinds of income generating programmes that provide elderly people with an opportunity to earn income by making productive use of their free time. Two are operated under the supervision of the Ministry of Health and Welfare — the Elderly Employment Centre and the Elderly Workshop — and three are operated under the supervision of the Ministry of Labour: the Older Workers' Bank, Older Workers' Job Selection and the Older Workers Employment Quota.

The Elderly Employment Centre links employers and elderly job seekers. The Elderly Workshop helps to set up workshops where elderly people can work together and receive remuneration for their work. The Older Workers Employment Promotion Law was enforced under the supervision of the Ministry of Labour in 1992. This law stipulates the establishment of the Older Workers' Bank, which is very similar to the Elderly

Employment Centre Program under the supervision of the Ministry of Health and Welfare, but which is particularly focused on those aged between 55 and 64. This law also stipulates that the government should identify and focus on jobs most appropriate to older workers, and should encourage employers to employ older workers, particularly in these jobs (Older Workers' Job Selection). In addition, this law recommends workplaces with more than 300 full time workers to hire older workers so that they comprise more than 3 per cent of the total number of workers (Older Workers Employment Quota). However, the non-compulsory nature of these requirements makes the law's recommendations unenforceable.

Retirement Benefit programme
This programme is compulsorily applicable to all workplaces by the provision of the law, even though it is not rigidly applied. The law requires employers, public or private, to pay each individual worker one month's salary per year into a retirement benefit fund, provided that the worker has been employed for more than one year. Therefore, any full-time worker who has worked for more than one year is eligible for Retirement Benefit (RB). The RB is paid as a lump sum when workers leave their workplaces on reaching the mandatory retirement age, or for other reasons. Currently, this programme is the principal income source for most retirees in Korea because the public pension has not yet matured.

Health care programmes

Health care cost payment programmes

Medical Insurance Programme.   The NHI pays for diagnosis, in-patient and out-patient treatment, operations, nursing, medication, and transport for treatment. For older persons the NHI covers all ambulatory and in-patient care on a year-round basis, but does not cover eye glasses, hearing aids, dentures and other prostheses. The payment level varies with the medical care system and the kind of treatment. The NHI pays 50–70 per cent of the fees for out-patient care and 80 per cent for in-patient care, while the patients themselves have to pay 20 per cent or more of the total medical fees. To be eligible for the NHI Programme, a person should be either the insured or a dependent family member of the insured.

The NHI scheme is financed by equal contributions from both employee and employer for those in workplaces, and by equal contributions from both the insured, and the government for rural community residents and the self-employed. The NHI scheme is administered by the National Health Insurance Corporation and its nationwide branches.

Medical Assistance Programme. The Medical Assistance programme (MA) covers not only NBLS recipients but also veterans, human cultural treasures, and disaster-stricken people. The MA scheme pays for the same categories of benefits as the MI scheme, but its payment level varies with the status of the recipient and the medical care system involved (primary and secondary). Deductible amounts are imposed on those who receive self-reliance benefits under the NBLS Programme (public assistance in income maintenance programmes). When they are unable to make payments, the state makes loans without interest with a reimbursement period of one to three years. This programme is financed by the contributions of central and local governments and the medical fees paid by recipients, and is administered under the auspices of the local governments. As of 2001, 3.5 per cent of all Koreans and 8.0 per cent of all those aged 65 and over were covered by this MA programme (Ministry of Health and Welfare Korea 2001*a*).

Health care services programmes
There are five health care service programmes: elderly health examinations, nursing homes, homes for the aged, visiting nurse and nursing hospital programmes. With the exception of elderly health examinations, all may be said to be long-term care services.

Elderly Health Examination Programme. The Elderly Health Examination (EHE) Programme was established by the Elderly Welfare Law of 1981 for the detection and prevention of diseases.

The state's provision is not compulsory and is subject to budgetary constraints.

Nursing Care Programme.   Nursing care services are available for those who need long-term care. Nursing homes are classified into five categories according to the fee-charging system and the nature of the illness: free nursing homes, low-fee charging nursing homes, full-fee charging nursing homes, free skilled nursing homes and full-fee charging skilled nursing homes. In 2001 there were 177 homes, comprising 96 free, 13 low-fee charging, 11 full-fee charging, 54 free skilled homes and 3 full-fee charging skilled homes. The Elderly Welfare Law Amendment of 1993 allows profit-making as well as non-profit organizations to run full-fee nursing homes, although at present all nursing homes are operated by non-profit organizations. Nursing home fees are not reimbursed by medical insurance.

Homes for the Aged Programme.   As mentioned above, institutional homes for the aged in Korea may have to be considered to be LTC facilities because there are many elderly people in homes for the aged who need long-term care. According to a survey of homes for the aged in 1999, about 60 per cent of elderly residents had problems in their ADL. As of 2000, there were 119 homes for the aged accommodating 5,694 elderly persons.

Geriatric Hospitals.   Geriatric hospitals were newly stipulated in the amendment to the Elderly Welfare Law of 1997. Accordingly, this category of hospital requires approval by the Ministry of Health and Welfare and, in 1999 there were 7 such geriatric hospitals.

Visiting Nurse Programme.   Visiting nurse services are not yet stipulated in the Elderly Welfare Law, but are stipulated in the Community Health Law and Medical Service Law. These services are regarded as one of the major community care services. They are provided by general hospitals, community health centres, the Korean Nurses Association and by community welfare centres although hospital-based and community health centre-based services are the major types. A majority of the users of visiting nurse services are older persons aged 60 and over (Whang et al. 1999).

Housing programmes

Korean housing policy for older persons can be divided in two parts according to the object of the policy: one for those who are residing in the community, and the other for those who are living in institutional settings.

According to the Elderly Welfare Law, all elderly welfare facilities are categorized into four groups: elderly housing welfare facilities, elderly medical welfare facilities, recreational facilities and home/community care facilities. Of these four categories, the housing welfare facility and the health care facility are related to the housing for older persons, housing facilities for the elderly, which accommodate elderly persons in relatively good health, are categorized into five subgroups: free homes for the aged, low-fee charging homes for the aged, full-fee charging homes for the aged, low-fee charging elderly welfare housing and full-fee charging welfare housing. The housing facility can be considered as a kind of congregate housing only for older persons. The health care facilities for the elderly are classified into six sub-groups: free nursing homes, low-fee charging nursing homes, full-fee charging nursing homes, free skilled nursing homes, full-fee charging skilled nursing homes and geriatric hospitals.

Of the five types of housing facilities defined under the Elderly Welfare Law, the low-fee charging and full-fee charging welfare housing systems for the aged may be treated as the general housing for older persons, and the other three types of older persons' housing facility may be treated as institutional housing.

Housing programmes for older persons living in the community
Despite the fact that the demand for housing designed for older persons is increasing, it could be said that there is no explicit housing policy for older Koreans living in the community. There

are several reasons for this (Choi 1999*a*). First of all, up to now, the overall housing shortage has been so serious that there has been little room to consider a housing policy aimed specifically at the elderly population. The provision of the Elderly Welfare Law that the state or the local government should facilitate the construction of houses appropriate for elderly people is ambiguous in terms of the government's responsibilities. Consequently, housing programmes in accordance with this provision have rarely been created. Since social welfare policy for older persons has focused mainly on institutional care, the government has not paid attention to the housing needs of elderly people living in the community.

The provisions stipulated in the Elderly Welfare Law are not, in fact, really concerned with housing for the majority of the elderly population, who are middle-and upper-class. Because the Elderly Welfare Law is mainly concerned with the welfare of poorer older persons only, the housing needs of the middle-and-upper-income elderly are neglected by the provisions of the Law.

Housing programmes for institutionalized older persons
It could be said that housing policy for older persons is formatted in terms of institutional types of housing — it deals with housing facilities and health care facilities. Because of the trends in social welfare policy for older persons that have placed more weight upon institutional care than on community care, housing policy for institutional care has been developed more in Korea than community care. The institutionalization rate of elderly Koreans is still very small, at only 0.3 per cent. Nevertheless, the increase in institutional types of elderly housing has been conspicuous over the past decade and the amount of institutional housing has doubled over the past ten years.

The Korean public's image of institutional type of housing is still relatively negative due to the poor services provided in those institutional settings which rely upon government's subsidies. This negative image seems to impede the development of such housing facilities, whether they are non-profit or for-profit and whether they are free or whether charges are levied.

Social service programmes

The needs and expectations of elderly Koreans have not only been elevated to higher levels but have also diversified to include, for example, personal help needs and social-psychological developmental needs amongst others. As family structures and functions have substantially changed, the family's need to strengthen its caring function has been increased and diversified. In spite of these changing needs, the number of social service programmes directed to meet the needs of the elderly population and their families are few in number.

There are two kinds of elderly welfare services providing social services for elderly persons: recreational programmes and community care programmes. Recreational programmes for older persons include senior centres, senior club houses, senior schools and senior resorts. The community care programmes include home-help services, adult day-care services, short-stay care services and visiting nurse services. These community care programmes are also available for long-term care for older persons residing in the community.

Recreational facilities for the elderly

Senior Centre Programme. The senior centre programmes are designed to provide a range of services concerning health improvement, adult education, recreation, counselling, information and guidance, amongst others. These centres are built with the assistance of central and local government, and their operational expenses are covered by local government. In 2001, there were 114 such elderly welfare centres being used regularly by about 330,000 elderly persons aged 60 and over.

Senior Club House Programme. Senior club houses established by voluntary donations from local people are the most generalized welfare facilities for the elderly in both urban and rural areas. Older Koreans come to the senior club houses for various leisure activities, such as watching television, reading newspapers and playing cards or chess, on a daily basis. However, organized programmes are seldom offered in the club houses, with most of the activities being casual (Choi 2000a). The government provides a small amount of money for operational expenses. In 2001, there were more than 40,000 club houses with members comprising about one-third who were aged 60 and over.

Senior School Programme.   The senior schools have been established by voluntary organizations, senior centres and community welfare centres to promote cultural, educational and recreational programmes for older persons. They are the second most generalized welfare facilities provided for elderly Koreans. As of 2001, there were about 600 schools for the elderly registered at the Ministry of Health and Welfare, with 957,000 elderly persons attending. Besides those registered, there are about 600 such schools which are not registered. Government financial assistance to schools for the elderly is meager and nominal. In addition to this type of school, some universities have recently opened life-long education classes for retirees. These programmes are becoming so popular that many higher educational institutions plan to open senior classes as well.

Senior Resort Facility Programme.   This programme aims to provide facilities for recreation and rest. Fees for the resort facilities are relatively expensive and the resorts are few in number. In 2001, there were six such facilities, used by an average of 5,000 elderly people each month.

Community care programmes

Home-Help Programme.   Home-help services are currently provided, free of charge, exclusively to elderly people receiving benefits under the NBLS. These services are provided by volunteers under the supervision of the service organizations. Home-help services include home-life support (such as grocery shopping and domestic cleaning), counselling and education (home-life supervision, training for improving ADL, education for handicapped elderly people and their caregivers), and arrangement of sponsors who can provide financial and/or emotional support for frail older persons. In 2001, about 35,000 volunteer home helpers were active, linked to 552 voluntary organizations. The government provides these voluntary organizations with financial assistance for recruiting, training and maintaining volunteers. However, as services are provided by volunteers, in most cases older persons cannot receive adequate services when they need them.

Adult Day-Care Programme.   Adult day-care programmes were somewhat unfamiliar to most elderly Koreans and their family members until recently. However, as the elderly population increases, demand has increased and continues to do so. As of 2001, there were 100 day-care centres operating at almost maximum capacity. Many elderly service centres, as well as community welfare agencies, have shown interest in opening more day-care programmes for older persons. Like many other services, these adult day-care programmes are also mainly provided only to older persons on low-incomes, for a small charge. Since paid adult day-care services are relatively underdeveloped, middle- and-upper class elderly people still do not have many opportunities to utilize such services.

Short-stay Care Programme.   Short-stay, respite services for older persons, which allow older persons to stay at nursing homes or elderly service centres in the community and be cared for a limited period (usually 2 to 45 full days per admission), are also provided (at 26 places in 2001). Fees are charged to users of these services. Like adult day-care services, short-stay respite-type services are not widely known to many Koreans. However, the demand for this type of service is increasing as more elderly people and their families understand the need for these services, particularly for the care of older persons suffering from dementia. These short-stay services, particularly those assisted by the government, are usually also provided only to the low-income elderly. Paid services are again relatively underdeveloped, despite the fact that paid community care services became possible upon the amendment of the Elderly Welfare Law of 1993.

Meal Delivery Programme.   This programme, instituted in 2000, is aimed at delivering lunches free of charge to those poor and low-income elderly who experience difficulties in the activities of daily living (ADL) and who are also recipients of the Elder-Respect Pension. Meals are prepared at the elder-respect restaurants, community welfare centres, senior centres, or schools, and are delivered to older persons by elderly volunteers, younger female volunteers and volunteers from religious organizations. The programme costs are born in equal share by the central and local governments (Ministry of Health and Welfare Korea 2001*b*).

Care of older persons

Care for older persons, in most cases, can be regarded as long-term care (LTC). This can be classified into informal and formal care, according to the nature of the providers. In most countries, whether developed or developing, informal care, which is very natural and in accordance with the principle of "ageing in place", is usually the first choice of older persons. Indeed, in the case of the United States, two-thirds to three-quarters of people aged 65 and over rely on only informal care, while one-quarter rely on both informal and formal care (Garner 1995; Evashwick 1996).

In Korea, almost all older persons today who need LTC are cared for by informal caregivers. There are a number of reasons for this. These include, amongst others, a lack of long-term care services; traditional values of filial piety and family responsibility; face-saving cultural attitudes of being reluctant to use services provided by non-familial persons; and a lack of understanding of in-home/community care services. According to survey research conducted on older persons in the community under LTC (Rhee et al 1999), elderly Koreans rarely use formal LTC services, as is shown in Table 3.6. Informal caregivers are most frequently a spouse (46 per cent), followed by daughters-in-law (31 per cent), daughters (8 per cent) and sons (8 per cent).

The phenomenon of under-utilization of formal LTC has been strongly influenced by traditional values of filial piety and the spirit of family responsibility for care of the elderly. The traditional value of filial piety seems to be sustained, but ways

TABLE 3.6

Korea: Long-term Care Service Utilization Rates for Older People under LTC

Services	Use Without Charge	Use With Charge	Do Not Use	Total
Home help	0.9	6.1	93.0	100.0
Adult day care	0.0	0.0	100.0	100.0
Short stay care	0.4	0.0	99.6	100.0
Visiting nurse	0.6	0.9	98.5	100.0
Nursing home	0.0	0.2	99.8	100.0
Elderly hospital	0.2	0.6	99.2	100.0

Source: Rhee (1999).

of realizing this value are changing, becoming more practical and reasonable. However, the values of familism and communalism associated with filial piety are withering away and, instead, individualism and the trend towards the nuclear family is developing and expanding. Thus, the individual is increasingly being thought of as more important than the family, or both the individual and the family are being thought as equally important. These value changes tend to weaken the consciousness of family support and care for older persons by the family and within the family. Though the consciousness of family responsibility for taking care of older parents has been weakened with these value changes, a majority of family caregivers still think that the family is the most responsible care provider. In the survey by Rhee et al (1999), about 63 per cent of the respondents cited the family as being the primary responsible care provider.

Characteristics of policies on ageing for older Koreans

This chapter has reviewed the policy development process, current policies and care services utilization. It is possible to identify a number of characteristics of ageing policies in Korea, in particular the philosophical bases of policy programmes, and the characteristics of programme structure in terms of eligibility criteria, coverage, financing and the delivery system.

Philosophical bases of policies

Social policies in Korea are based on perspectives of "economic growth then distribution", reactive development and ageism, and the value of filial piety. Over the past 40 years, since the early 1960s, when the first economic development plan was implemented, strategies of social development have been overwhelmingly oriented towards economic development. Hence, fortunately or unfortunately, those Korean government bureaucrats who have held the most significant positions in policy-making have promoted the viewpoint of "economic growth then distribution".

Almost all of the social welfare programmes have been developed as piecemeal reactions to problems that have already occurred. Social welfare policies in general in Korea have therefore been reactive, short-term and of a piecemeal nature, and have not really considered a mid- and long-term perspective. Despite the fact that there exists little or no evidence to support the notion that productivity declines with ageing (as against the opposing view, that older workers can sometimes do equally well or better than their younger counterparts), the prejudiced ("ageist") belief that older persons are vulnerable and physically and mentally frail, and thus that their productivity declines with age, is prevalent in Korean society (Choi 1999*b*). This prejudice seems to have been part and parcel of the theoretical bases which negatively affect retirement and re-employment policies for elderly Koreans.

The traditional value of filial piety, which emphasizes family responsibility for the economic support of elderly people and the provision of care and services to them by their own family members living with them, still firmly underpins many of the social policies for older persons in Korea. In a modern welfare state, the emphasis on family responsibility based on the value of filial piety can make the state's responsibility minimal and can thus deter the development of state welfare provisions.

Filial piety can be dealt with at both the familial and the societal level. One of the most important bases for filial piety is the wish to repay one's parents for their love and care (Choi 1982, 1996). Therefore, one of the motivations for *individuals* to show filial piety at the familial level is to provide economic support and direct care services to parents in order to repay them for their love and care. One of the motivations for *the state* to practise filial piety at the societal level , in the form of welfare provisions, is to repay older persons for their contributions to society or to the state. Filial piety has traditionally been emphasized at the familial level, but not at the societal level. As a result, emphasizing the practice of filial piety merely at the familial level greatly hinders the development of formal LTC services at the state level.

Together with this continuance of filial piety, the perspective of family responsibility may contribute to the maintenance of face-saving attitudes towards caring for elderly parents. Accordingly, most Koreans still think it shameful to have their parents cared for by non-familial members and to have them institutionalized in homes for the aged or in nursing homes.

The concept of LTC and care of elderly parents by non-familial members and institutions is a relatively new concern, and presents a challenge to both families and the state. LTC is becoming a new challenge to the family in that it causes conflicts between the need for reasonable decision-making and prevalent face-saving cultural attitudes towards caregiving. LTC is becoming a new challenge to the state in that it is testing the state's capability to develop LTC policies.

Characteristics of the policy programme structures

Eligibility criteria
The eligibility criteria of policy programmes seem to be based on the residual perspective of social welfare, and show a lack of consideration for the difficulties of the current elderly generation. Though a minimum standard of living in terms of income maintenance is to be guaranteed with the legislation of the National Basic Livelihood Security Law of 1999, social services are in most cases focused on the low-income class and there exist few programmes for the middle-and upper-income class to utilize.

The National Pension (NP) Programme covering more than 90 per cent of all working Koreans did not consider those retirees who had already reached the pensionable age of 60 at the time of its inception (1988). The Elder-Respect Pension instituted to compensate for their unequal treatment provides such small amounts in terms of benefits that it may not be enough to provide a sufficient income for these pensioners' retirement life. In addition, re-employment policies are not well implemented because of the loose stipulations of the Elderly Welfare Law and the Older Workers Employment Promotion Law, and government's limited assistance with these re-employment policies. Hence, older people who are healthy and have accumulated occupational knowledge and skills throughout their working life rarely have opportunities to participate meaningfully in social or volunteer activities. Thus most of the elderly generation are caught in "roleless roles" and a vicious circle of negative images of their competence.

It is taken for granted that the priority target group in social welfare should be the poor but, as people's living standards rise and population ageing advances, the scope of the target group needs to be expanded to include middle-income class people. LTC needs arise regardless of income class. Particularly since LTC needs and problems have been more and more visible over the past ten years, paid or fee-charging LTC services need to be developed for those in the middle and upper socio-economic groups. Currently, few services are available for these middle- and upper-class elderly people.

As the lengthening of life expectancy continues, dependent life in later old age is becoming more common among older persons (OECD 1997). The LTC needs of older persons should therefore be met with the planned development of formal statutory services and informal care services.

Coverage and level of benefits
Policy programmes in Korea can be also characterized as having limited coverage, low levels of benefits and focusing on institutional care. Some important benefits in health care and social service programmes for older persons are lacking: expenses for long-term are not paid from medical insurance; visiting nurse services have not yet been instituted as a statutory community care service for older persons; and several housing

services need to be added, such as supplying rental housing and housing designed for the convenience of older persons. The level of benefits of many policy programmes is not adequate to maintain quality of life beyond the minimum. For example, the amount of the Elder-Respect Pension is too small to be of much help in covering living expenses, and government assistance to institutional care is also not sufficient to maintain quality services. In addition, the proportion of the national budget allocated to community care in 2001 was less than one-tenth that allocated to institutional care. This attests to the focus on institutional care in the national policies.

Most LTC services subsidized by the government (free and low fee-charging services in both institutional and community care) are poor or substandard in terms of quality. LTC policies still rely largely on institutional care. In most welfare states, welfare benefits tend to be provided to individuals after a breakdown in family functions rather than to support the family before breakdown. Such a policy has resulted in an increase in an institutionalized population and in ineffective and inefficient care services. Current community care programmes are limited to only three kinds: home-help services, adult day-care services and short-stay care (respite) services.

Few older persons use community care services (Table 3.6) and the occupancy rate of institutions is about 71 per cent. The present capacity of institutional care is about 20,000 and that of community care is also about 20,000. Although existing LTC services are not well utilized, present capacity is far below normatively estimated needs.

Currently there exists no formal statutory service for family caregivers except for one self-supportive family caregiver group. It is therefore not surprising that many family caregivers of older people with dementia suffer anxiety, anger, stress, lack of sleep and chronic fatigue (Kwon 1994). Housing designed for older persons to live more independently without others' help, or with little assistance from others, may enhance the effectiveness of LTC. However, policies do not require the housing to be specially designed for the convenience and needs of elderly people.

Finance

In terms of finance, policy programmes for older persons could be characterized as receiving low levels of government expenditure, lack of assistance from the community, and with an underdevelopment of services for middle- and upper-class elderly people. Government budgets for elderly welfare have been relatively small compared to Korea's GDP and the national budget for social welfare. The budget for social welfare has increased in Korea, but it still remains at less than 5 per cent of the national budget and less than 1 per cent of GDP. Although the welfare budget for older persons has steadily increased, it remained at less than 5 per cent of the social welfare budget until 1999.

Most voluntary social service organizations are heavily subsidized by the government, but subsidies are not sufficient to provide good quality services to elderly clients. Therefore, while there is much room for an increase in government assistance, voluntary organizations also need to secure a substantial amount of funds from the general public in order to improve and develop services in response to the emerging needs of older persons. There are few social service programmes for people whose income is above the poverty line. The Elderly Market, (ie products or services consumed by older persons in the market), which could be one way to finance and develop various services to respond to the needs of the middle- and upper-class elderly people, remains relatively underdeveloped.

Currently, there is no explicit financial programme for older persons or their families to pay for the costs of LTC. The existing National Health Insurance and Medical Assistance was not created for LTC, but to cure acute diseases, and social service funds are also not designed to pay for elderly persons' LTC costs. Private health insurance is a potential alternative to public LTC insurance — indeed, several types of private health insurance or disease-specific insurance to cover medical expenses have been developed, but these cover expenses for only a limited period of time. The government does not provide any special tax deduction incentives to those covered by private health insurance, and so people are not encouraged to subscribe such health insurance.

The delivery system

The delivery system of policy programmes is fused with many ministries other than the Ministry of Health and Welfare, and it lacks quality manpower and autonomy among voluntary service organizations. Since the delivery system for social welfare services is fused with the general administrative system, it is very hard for policy planning and service delivery to be conducted in a professional manner and to utilize people with professional expertise and knowledge of social welfare (Choi 2000*a*, 2000*b*). Because government subsidies provide almost all of the budgets of voluntary organizations, they are under the supervision of the public social service delivery systems. Therefore, it could be said that the planning and development of the service programmes of most voluntary organizations lacks in many aspects sufficient autonomy from government control.

Most institutions for the elderly tend to be of a large size, accommodating more than 100 residents. Conditions and terms for government subsidies indirectly contribute to the trend to larger scale institutions. Large size institutions may be good for economies of scale but they are very likely to lose the benefit of providing a home-like environment, and to together with other disadvantages that come with over-large facilities. The minimum numbers of medical staff and para-medical staff are also thought to be sub-standard and, with the number of qualified staff involved, it is very difficult to achieve sustainable high quality of services. Personnel shortages and a failure to train workers in the skills required for dealing with social welfare, particularly gerontology, has kept the quality of services provided to the elderly by both the public and voluntary sectors relatively low. For example,there are no licensed care workers (as exist for example in Japan) to take care of older persons with problems in their ADL.

Future prospects for policy development

The future environment in which welfare policies for older persons will be formulated seems to make the government facilitate further development by expanding the range of beneficiaries, creating more benefit categories, increasing government expenditure and improving the service delivery system. However, some of the major barriers to policy development involve the philosophical bases underpinning current policies, and these may be harder to change. Indeed, all these philosophical bases are in fact related to the government's reluctance to allocate more funds from other budget heads to social welfare programmes. In anticipating the development of government policy for older persons, two levels in the government's position have to be considered: that of the particular ministry involved, and that of coordination of that ministry with the Ministry of Planning and Budget or with the prime minister.

The Ministry of Health and Welfare fully recognizes the importance of policy development for older persons and has had several mid-term and long-term policy development plans. However, these plans do not include methods of financing to secure the budget and, without a budget plan corresponding to policy programmes and financing methods, the policy plan cannot be properly implemented. Policy plans made at the prime ministerial and presidential level, even without budget plans and financing methods, tend to be relatively well implemented. However, plans designed at the ministerial level, which usually do not have budget plans approved by the Ministry of Planning and Budget, have not usually been well implemented, or have been only partially implemented. It is usually very difficult for policy plans formulated at the ministerial level to gain approval from the Ministry of Planning and Budget in order to finance the policy programmes.

There are two other plans for policy development. One is the Mid-and Long-term Plan for Health and Welfare Policies for the Elderly, set up by the Ministry of Health and Welfare in 1999; the other is the New Millennium Welfare Vision 2010, a long-term plan for health and welfare policies lasting until 2010. However, since both plans do not have budget plans approved by the Ministry of Planning and Budget, it is likely to be very difficult for the ministry to implement these plans.

Nevertheless, it seems inevitable that the general environment surrounding policies for older persons will necessitate the government developing policies for the elderly from a longer-term perspective in the future. The belief in "economic growth then distribution" will wither away as economic growth continues and, consequently, GDP per capita increases. When this occurs, a substantial degree of policy development should then be possible.

With the establishment of the Long-term Care Policy Planning Committee under the Ministry of Health and Welfare in 2000, LTC policies began to be officially discussed at the government level. As noted earlier, the term "LTC" began to be used from the late 1990s, though its meaning has been understood for more than ten years. There may be several factors stimulating the official discussion of LTC at government level. For instance, since the mid-1990s, there have been many debates on preventive measures against rapid population ageing and on Korean society becoming an "ageing society" in which the proportion of older persons aged 65 and over is beyond 7 per cent but under 14 per cent. Elsewhere in the region, Japan's enactment of a LTC Law in 1997 and its introduction in April 2000 may have stimulated Korean concerns about LTC and its financial implications. Whatever the cause, the term LTC is recognized and concern about LTC policy development is becoming an important issue in Korea. In response to the recommendation of the LTC Policy Planning Committee (LTC Policy Planning Committee, Ministry of Health and Welfare, Korea 2000), the government conducted an LTC Needs Survey and developed ADL/IADL measurement scales.

Many conspicuous factors over the past ten years have made it necessary to develop LTC policies from a long-term perspective. Major factors include demographic ageing and rapid growth of the oldest-old population, deterioration of traditional values, changes in family structure (particularly caused by rising trends in older persons living separately from their adult children), increasing medical expenditure requirements of older persons, and increases in the proportion of frail and disabled elderly people due to physical and mental ageing (Ministry of Health and Welfare Korea 2000c).

As elsewhere, fiscal matters have also been important. For example, in 2001, it was revealed that there was a great deficit in National Health Insurance funds. This deficit seems to have been aggravated by the integration of existing medical insurances into one system (National Health Insurance) and the new medical care system designed to strictly separate the roles of doctors and pharmacists, which began in July 2000. This surprised Koreans. A comprehensive plan on measures to solve the deficit problems reported by the Minister of Health and Welfare identified one of the major causes for the rise in medical expenses as an increase in hospital visits by older persons and also as population ageing (Ministry of Health and Welfare Korea 2001c). Therefore, the government is considering public LTC insurance from a mid-term or long-term perspective. In addition to the LTC insurance plan, the government proposes to increase long-term care facilities and to activate visiting nurse services. Since these LTC-related plans are a stated promise by the government to Korean citizens, the probability of proceeding with them as planned seems to be very high.

It is nevertheless known that many of government's mid- and long-term plans have not been properly implemented. This experience of not seeing plans implemented as proposed makes the public somewhat uncertain about the possible future implementation of LTC-related plans. Therefore, citizens' groups and gerontologists, as well as interested elderly groups, need to monitor government actions and to apply pressure on government bureaucrats and the political parties concerned to ensure implementation.

Conclusion

The issues surrounding ageing in Korea are perceived as a new concern and as a challenge that has never before been experienced. With the demographic ageing of Korea's population, LTC is emerging as an important feature. Indeed, if the experience of developed countries is considered, from a long-term perspective, producing appropriate LTC policies is both necessary and proper. The necessity for such policies in Korea is becoming ever more evident due to the government's persistent economic growth-oriented strategies for national development, bureaucrats' erroneous perspectives on issues related to ageing, the lack of attention to, and the government's belated responses to, the problem and, associated with this, the government's unrealistic fears of welfare expansion. All these factors function as barriers to the development of social welfare policies for older persons that should be harmonized with the degree of socio-economic development that has been achieved in Korean society over the past forty years.

In reality, it may be difficult to expect a substantial degree of policy development in the near future, but it is not sensible to sit and wait until the proper time comes. Korea needs to seek out strategies to advance social welfare policies for older persons as soon as possible. Important questions remain. How can social welfare policies for older persons be advanced to match socio-economic development? What strategies will help to achieve harmony between socio-economic development and social welfare for older persons in the future? This chapter concludes by suggesting some strategies to balance socio-economic development and social welfare development for older persons.

Some, indeed any, influence on the formulation of political party programmes is needed. It can be particularly opportune and effective to influence policy-making when presidential and general elections are about to take place. A strategy that could influence politicians through both persuasion and education is to hold regular study or discussion meetings with congressmen with regard to general or specific agendas. Gerontologists may use and participate in the citizen's movement to influence legislation for social welfare programmes for older persons. Indeed, many Koreans believe that the NBLS law was a victory for citizens' organizations. Another strategy to influence policy-making is to organize a national association of older persons which can exercise political power in policy-making.

Ageing is regarded by many in Korea as a set of problems that, while they may challenge contemporary Korean society, could act as an accelerator to build up a viable welfare state. This requires the government to change its arguably outmoded perceptions, which to now have acted as a safeguard for economic development but which have also built barriers to the development of social welfare. The Korean government, benefiting from the experience of other advanced countries, could now take positive steps to develop social welfare policies for older persons. This will be one of the most significant components for the building of a Korean welfare state.

4

Ageing in Malaysia
A Review of National
Policies and Programmes

Ong Fon Sim

Introduction

Malaysia's population is not currently particularly elderly, although this will change over the next two decades or so. The 2000 Census showed that 6.2 per cent, 1.452 million people, were aged 60 or over, but demographic ageing is occurring and, by the year 2020, 9.5 per cent of the country's population will be aged 60 years and over. In accordance with the United Nations World Assembly on Ageing held in Vienna in 1982, at which the age of 60 years and over was adopted for deliberating issues on ageing, Malaysia has also adopted this demarcation in formulating and implementing plans for its senior citizens. However, the present retirement age of 56 seems to suggest that the threshold for ageing locally is felt to begin at 56 years of age.

Malaysia has been experiencing improved health, longer life expectancy, low mortality as well as declining fertility. The combination of all of these has brought about a change in the demographic profile of the country's population. The age structure for the past four censuses (in 1970, 1980, 1991 and 2000) shows that the proportion of younger age groups (15 years and below) is decreasing, while the proportion of elderly is on the rise. The median age was 17.4 in 1970, 21.9 in 1991, 23.6 in 2000 and is projected to increase to 27.1 in the year 2020. Within a period of thirty years (from 1991 to 2020), the median age will have increased on average by 1.7 per decade. The old-age dependency ratio is expected to increase to 15.7 in 2020 from 10.5 in 1970. This is high compared to other ASEAN countries such as Indonesia (10.1), Thailand (13.4), and the Philippines (9.0), although Singapore has a dependency rate of 23.9 (and Japan's ratio of 41.5). Over a period of 50 years, the median age of the Malaysian population will increase by 10, and the old-age dependency ratio by 5 (Department of Statistics, Malaysia 1998). By the year 2020, Malaysia will be a mature society with 9.5 per cent of its population aged 60 and above. Although the rate of increase of its population ageing is slower than that of countries such as China and Singapore, the increase in the proportion of older persons will make it impossible for the government to ignore the social and economic impacts of population ageing.

This chapter reviews Malaysia's national policy on ageing and long-term care, and aims to:

- Review of the picture of ageing in Malaysia from the perspectives of social security, health, community care and social services
- Review policies and programmes for older persons, including long-term care
- Examine the main features of these policies and programmes
- Examine the role of civil society or NGOs in providing inputs into the formulation of policy, and
- Discuss the likely developments with respect to policies and programmes for older persons.

This chapter relies heavily on secondary data as well as discussions and interviews with experts in specific areas such as social security, health care and social services. As issues concerning older persons are inherently multi-disciplinary in nature, data and information were obtained from different ministries and departments. Data were drawn from the population censuses of 1980, 1991 and 2000, although a disadvantage is that the census does not cover details such as older persons' health status, their contributions to society and family and their involvement in social and charitable activities. Where data gaps exist, they are supplemented as available with research findings from smaller studies of limited geographical coverage.

Profile of Malaysia's ageing population

Within Malaysia, the rate of growth of senior citizens shows spatial variations, with rural areas containing a larger proportion of the elderly population compared with urban areas. In 2000, the percentage of the elderly population in rural areas was 7.5, compared with 6.5 in 1991. The urban proportions registered a mere 0.1 per cent growth rate during the period 1991–2000 (Table 4.1). The slow rate of growth of the elderly population in urban areas is due partly to the out-migration of the young rural population to the urban areas in search of employment and education opportunities, as well as the influx of foreign labour into Malaysia.

Demographic Variations

Ethnic variations
Due to inter-group socio-economic differences, as well as the influence of historical, institutional, and economic factors, experiences of demographic transition vary in both intensity and timing among Malaysia's three major ethnic groups (*Bumiputra* Malays, Chinese and Indians). Demographic ageing is significantly more advanced among the Chinese than in the other two groups (Table 4.1). In 1991, 7.6 per cent of the Chinese were elderly, a percentage much higher than that among the Malays (5.4 per cent) and Indians (5.4 per cent). In 2000, the percentage of elderly people among the Chinese has increased further to 8.8 per cent (Table 4.1). This growth in demographic ageing is due to the low mortality and longer life expectancy among the Chinese, as well as a low fertility rate that substantially reduces the size of the young population. This combined effect has been evident for much longer for the Chinese than in the other ethnic groups.

TABLE 4.1

Malaysia: Persons Aged 60 and Above by Ethnic Group and Residence 1991, 2000 and 2020

Ethnic Group	1991 Per cent Urban	Rural	Total	Number ('000)	2000 Per cent Urban	Rural	Total	Number ('000)	2020ᵃ Number ('000)	Per cent
Malaysian citizens										
Bumiputera	3.5	6.6	5.4	552.1	3.7	7.7	5.6	804.2		7.9
Chinese	7.4	8.0	7.6	348.4	8.4	11.3	8.8	501.0		14.4
Indian	5.8	4.8	5.4	71.1	5.6	5.5	5.6	93.9		10.4
Others	4.5	8.0	6.9	39.5	3.8	6.1	4.6	12.5		8.3
Total	5.4	6.7	6.0	1,012.1	5.6	7.9	6.4	1,411.5		9.5
Non-Malaysian	3.7	1.9	2.7	20.2	3.6	1.9	2.9	40.2		9.5
Total	**5.3**	**6.5**	**5.9**	**1,032.3**	**5.4**	**7.5**	**6.2**	**1,451.7**		**9.5**
Number ('000)	470.8	561.5	1,032.3		785.3	666.4	1,451.7		3,209.8	

ᵃ Figures for 2020 are projections.

Source: Department of Statistics, Malaysia (1998, 2001).

This trend is expected to continue, and the proportion of elderly Chinese is projected to be around 14.4 per cent by the year 2020, at which time the proportion of Indian senior citizens is projected to be 10.4 whilst that of the Malays will be 7.9 per cent.

Gender differences

Although demographic ageing appears inevitable, the situations facing males and females can be very different. Table 4.2 indicates the decline in the sex ratio among older Malaysians. In 1970, there were more elderly males than females (108.4), but the ratio had dropped to 89.6 by 1991, before rising marginally again to 91.4 in 2000 (Table 4.2). Among the major ethnic groups, demographic changes in the Indian community are the most marked, in that the male–female ratio was 216.6 in 1970, 86.8 in 2000 and is expected to drop to 74.8 in 2020. This means that there will be far more female elderly persons compared to males, and the implications for social security will be profound. Among the *Bumiputras* (indigenous people), the ratio of male to female elderly persons was 102.8 in 1970, which dropped to 90.7 in 2000

TABLE 4.2

Malaysia: Sex Ratio Among People Aged 60 and Above by Age Group and Ethnic Group, 1970–2020

	1970	1980	1991	2000	2020*
Age group	*Sex ratio*	*Sex ratio*	*Sex ratio*	*Sex ratio*	*Sex ratio*
Total (60+)	108.4	97.2	89.6	91.4	85.2
60–74	112.1	98.2	91.7	94.7	89.0
75+	89.5	93.4	82.2	79.2	85.2
Ethnic group[b]					
Bumiputra	102.8	99.3	91.6	90.7	83.8
Chinese	102.8	86.3	79.4	91.5	87.3
Indians	216.6	163.5	114.3	86.8	74.8

[a] Projection.
[b] The classification of ethnic groups for 1970 and 1980 differs from the classification used in 1991 onwards. The main ethnic groups include only Malaysian citizens since the 1991 Census, whereas previously the classification included both citizens and non-citizens.
Source: Department of Statistics, Malaysia (1998, 2001).

and is expected to decrease further to 83.8 in 2020. The Chinese community experienced a similar situation in which the ratio was 102.8 in 1970, 91.5 in 2000 and 87.3 in 2020. Demographic ageing in Malaysia as elsewhere seems to skew towards more females, especially among the Indians compared to the other two ethnic groups, suggesting that problems associated with widowhood will be more serious among this ethnic group. The trend seems to suggest the feminization of ageing in the future, with concomitant challenges to family care and costs.

Marital status

Table 4.3 shows that in 1991, almost one in three senior citizens was classified as widowed. There was a strong contrast between elderly widowed males, who constituted only 12 per cent of male elderly population, whereas widowed females constituted over half (51 per cent) of the female elderly group. By 2000, the percentage of widowed males had dropped marginally to 11.4 per cent, whereas the percentage of female widowed dropped

TABLE 4.3

Malaysia: Older Persons' Marital Status by Sex and Age Group, 1991 and 2000 (percentages)

Marital Status	Male			Female			Total		
	60–74	75+	Total	60–74	75+	Total	60–74	75+	Total
1991									
Never married	2.1	2.0	2.0	1.5	1.5	1.5	1.8	1.7	1.8
Currently married	87.4	71.1	84.1	49.7	24.0	44.0	67.7	45.3	62.9
Widowed	9.3	24.8	12.4	45.2	70.2	50.7	28.0	49.8	32.8
Divorced/ Permanently separated	1.3	2.1	1.4	3.6	4.3	3.8	2.5	3.3	2.7
Total	100.0	100.0	100.0	100.0	100.0	100.0	100.0	100.0	100.0
2000									
Never married	2.2	1.9	2.2	2.1	1.5	1.9	1.8	1.7	2.0
Currently married	88.3	73.4	85.6	56.3	27.5	50.2	61.4	47.8	67.1
Widowed	8.6	23.5	11.4	39.6	68.7	45.8	35.3	48.7	29.4
Divorced/ Permanently separated	0.79	1.16	0.9	2.01	2.4	2.1	1.6	1.8	1.5
Total	100.0	100.0	100.0	100.0	100.0	100.0	100.0	100.0	100.0

Source: Department of Statistics, Malaysia (1998, 2001).

substantially to 45.8 per cent. Overall, a far greater percentage of males were married and the differences in marital status became even more evident in the oldest-old age groups, where 71.1 and 73.4 per cent (for 1991 and 2000) of males were married compared to only 24.0 and 27.5 per cent of females.

Education

As in many other countries of the Asia–Pacific region, the present cohort of Malaysian older persons are not well educated (1991 Census) due to the limited educational opportunities during the nation's economic development in the early decades of the twentieth century. Some 63 per cent of older persons had received no schooling at all, although this represented an improvement on the figures in 1970 and 1980, in which those with no education represented, respectively, 75 and 73 per cent (Table 4.4). This trend is not expected to continue, as education has become widely available and future cohorts of elderly people will be better educated. Assuming that the present cohort of population aged between 35 and 54 is to move into the aged group and assuming that the present educational achievements of these people remain the same, by 2020 the educational profile of this cohort of senior citizens will show most to have some education, with 6 per cent having tertiary education and only 20 per cent having received no schooling.

TABLE 4.4

Malaysia: Education Levels of Older Persons, 1970–2020 (percentages)

	1970	1980	1991	2020[a]
No schooling	75.0	73.2	63.1[b]	20.3
Primary	22.3	23.1	31.5	45.5
Lower secondary	1.3	1.8	2.4	15.1
Upper secondary	1.2	1.5	2.1	13.2
Tertiary	0.3	0.4	0.9	5.9
Total	100.0	100.0	100.0[b]	100.0

[a] Estimates.
[b] Includes 1 per cent of cases where the educational level was unknown.
Source: Department of Statistics, Malaysia (1998).

Educational attainment by gender shows that a much lower percentage of females were educated compared to males during this period, consistent with the past social cultural environment, which accorded preference for boys in education. According to the 1991 Census, almost half (47 per cent) of elderly males had received basic schooling compared to only 18 per cent of females.

Economic activity

Although it is recognized that labour force participation generally declines as age increases, the decline that Malaysia experienced between the 1980 and 1991 censuses was significant, not only in terms of percentage decline but also in absolute numbers. Table 4.5 indicates that labour force participation rate (LFPR) declined from 39.1 in 1980 to 25.6 in 1991. In absolute numbers, the total number decreased from 290,000 in 1980 to 263,000 in 1991 (Department of Statistics Malaysia, 1998). In the case of females, the decrease has been even more significant, with a decline of almost 50 per cent from 1980 to 1991. Even among the young older group (aged 60 to 64), the LFPR showed a decline from 69 per cent to 56 per cent among males and from 27 per cent to 16 per cent among females.

TABLE 4.5

Malaysia: Labour Force Participation Rates (LFPR) of Older Persons by Sex and Age Group, 1970, 1980 and 1991

Year and Age	Male	Female	Total
1970	54.7	18.4	37.3
1980	56.8	21.8	39.1
1991	41.9	10.9	25.6
1980			
60–64	69.4	26.7	47.7
65+ years	49.7	19.0	34.2
1991			
60–64	55.6	16.1	35.2
65+ years	33.8	8.1	20.1

Source: Department of Statistics, Malaysia (1998).

The economic activities of the present elderly cohort still mirror the past economic structure of Malaysia, in which agriculture was the major sector providing the greatest number of jobs and 62 per cent of older persons worked in the agricultural sector (1991 Census).

Living arrangements
Development in Malaysia has been accompanied by changes in family structure in which smaller family size and a preference for nuclear families are replacing the extended family structure and larger families. Migration of the younger population to the urban areas and the growth in female labour-force participation have all had an effect on the family as caregivers for older persons. In addition to having to cope with self-care, some older persons who remain in the rural areas also shoulder the responsibility of caring for their grandchildren. Sometimes, the pressures on them are compounded by changes in the life cycle, such as the loss of a spouse or a decline in health, that affects older persons directly.

Table 4.6 shows that in Malaysia, the average household size decreased from 5.2 in 1980 to 4.8 in 1991. Although the nuclear

TABLE 4.6
Malaysia: Average Household Size and Rate of Household Types by Stratum, 1980 and 1991

Household Type	1980	1991
Average household size		
Total households	5.2	4.8
Nuclear family households	4.9	4.8
Extended family households	7.1	6.5
Rate (per cent)		
Nuclear family households	55.2	59.9
Urban	50.4	58.7
Rural	57.7	61.1
Extended family households	27.8	26.4
Urban	29.3	27.2
Rural	27.0	25.7

Source: Department of Statistics, Malaysia (1998).

family household size remained fairly constant, the extended family household size has decreased from 7.1 to 6.5 between 1980 and 1991. The proportion of nuclear families showed an increase, while extended family types declined, albeit very gradually.

In terms of marital status and gender, in 1991, almost 87 per cent of older persons were part of nuclear family households and were still married (Department of Statistics Malaysia, 1998). As noted above, almost all males were married whereas one in four females were widowed. Among extended family households, 58.8 per cent of older persons were married, indicating intergenerational living arrangements. Analysis by gender shows that almost 54 per cent of females were widows living with married children, whereas only 15 per cent of males were widowed. Tan et al. (1999) found that more than 25 per cent of older persons co-resided with their spouse and children and/or with others, indicating an extended-family type of living arrangement. The Malays had a higher incidence of nuclear families compared to the Chinese and Indians.

National policy for older persons

Until 1995, there was no specific policy for older persons in Malaysia. At best, policies or programmes catering to the needs of older persons were largely incorporated into overall social welfare policy development. The National Welfare Policy promulgated in 1990 identifies older persons as one of its many target groups. Although this is the first ever specific public sector effort recognizing the need to care for older persons, families and communities are encouraged or expected to continue to provide care to older persons. The principle is that institutional support should be the last resort.

In 1995, the Government formulated the National Policy for the Elderly aimed at: "creating a society of elderly people who are contented and possess a high sense of *self worth* and *dignity*, by *optimizing their self potential* and ensuring that they enjoy *every opportunity* as well as [the] *care and protection* [of] members of their family, society and nation" (Government of Malaysia 1996, p. 571, emphasis added). Specifically, the policy has the objectives of upgrading the dignity and self-worth of senior citizens within the family, society and nation, and of improving the potential of older persons so that they can continue to be productive in national development. The policy also aims at encouraging the provision of facilities for older persons so as to ensure care and protection for them. In line with these objectives, several action plans have been initiated and six sub-committees established under a National Senior Citizens Policy Technical Committee set up by the Social Welfare Department in July 1996. These six sub-committees were social and recreational; health; education, religion and training; housing; research, and publicity. Under each of these sub-committees, many activities and programmes have been started and many more are planned. Various ministries and departments are involved in the action plans and activities for older persons, but the agency that oversees all matters is the Department of Social Welfare, in the Ministry of National Unity and Social Development.

Although the policy has been a great step forward in preparing Malaysia for a transition to an ageing society, the 1999 Malaysian Plan of Action does not adequately cover employment and income security. The emphasis of the policy appears to be on social aspects, although these do of course contribute towards the overall well-being of older persons.

National policy on long-term care (LTC)

As noted in Chapter 1, long-term care may be defined as care delivered to individuals who are dependent on others for assistance with the basic tasks necessary for physical, mental, and social functioning over sustained periods of time. The goal of LTC is usually to allow recipients to function at the highest level of autonomy possible. At the institutional level, a stay at an institution for three months or more is typically described as long-term. However, besides institutional care, the vast majority of those requiring LTC depend on informal sources of support — family and friends, as well as community care (Phillips 2000). The family often remains the primary caregiver to frail older persons.

Malaysia does not have a national policy specifically on long-term care, although some preliminary discussions had taken place prior to the Asian economic crisis of 1997–98. However, the absence of a policy does not reflect a total absence of regulations, infrastructure and facilities for the provision of services necessary to support LTC. From the regulatory perspective, the Care Centre Act 1993, and Care Centre Regulations 1994 exist to govern the minimum standards that protect the interests of older persons in Malaysia. The Private Healthcare Facilities and Services Act 1998 stipulates guidelines and regulations specifically for nursing homes. It might be speculated that the future direction will be towards the formalization of a policy on LTC, although this is not to be expected in the foreseeable future.

Social security and economic well-being

In Malaysia, formal social protection includes the Employees Provident Fund (EPF) set up in 1951, the Social Security Organization (SOCSO) established in 1969, the Government Pension Scheme for Civil Servants, the Old Age Benefit Scheme for the Armed Forces, and private sector provident and pension funds. These different schemes provide protection for different contingencies such as disability, as in the case of SOCSO, old age (pensions and the EPF) and death. While these schemes provide coverage for the formal sector, the provision is not mandatory for those in the informal sector, which is substantial in Malaysia. Although the EPF is extended to the self-employed on a voluntary contribution basis, the participation rate is low. Therefore, those in the informal sector have to rely on savings, drawing down on past wealth and financial support from children to provide them with income security in their old age. Due to the lack of data on the informal sector, it is difficult to assess the extent of protection available to older persons in this sector.

The two major schemes in Malaysia are often referred to as "pillars": Pillar 1, pension, is based on defined benefits, and Pillar 2, EPF, is a defined contribution system, in which benefits depend on the assets in the individual's account at retirement (Fox and Palmer 2001).

Pension

Pension is a non-contributory social security scheme for government employees. Pensions expenditure is wholly borne by the federal government through annual allocation from the federal budget, and is a pay-as-you-go plan. An employee who has served at least 10 years is entitled to receive a life-long monthly pension upon retirement. The amount receivable by an employee who has completed at least 25 years of service is half of the last drawn salary. This scheme serves not only as security for old age but is also designed to provide financial assistance to the dependents of those in government service in the event that the government employee dies in service or after retirement. It also provides compensation to officers who die or are forced to retire due to injuries or sickness received in the course of performing their official duties. The types of retirement benefits offered in the pension scheme include a service pension and a service gratuity, a lump sum payment granted upon retirement. The other type of benefit is in the form of a derivative pension and a gratuity, granted to the dependents of permanent and confirmed officers who die in service. It is a safety net for widowed spouses and is particularly beneficial in providing for females, who generally experience a higher incidence of widowhood. However, in terms of coverage, fewer than 1 per cent of the population is protected.

Employee Provident Fund (EPF)

The EPF began as a simple, easy to understand and easy to administer scheme that allows workers an avenue to save. It is a trust fund established under the EPF Ordinance, 1951, (amended to the EPF Act in 1991). The EPF is a defined contribution plan based on a prescribed rate of contributions by employers and employees, accumulated as savings in a personal account with full withdrawal upon retirement. The scheme is mandatory for those in the formal sector, but it also allows those who are self-employed to contribute towards the fund. This flexibility is aimed at encouraging savings for old age. The rate of contributions is

12 per cent and 9 per cent for employers and employees respectively, regardless of the age of the employee.

The EPF is structured into three types of accounts: namely Account I (60 per cent), Account II (30 per cent) and Account III (10 per cent). Each account is designed to serve the different needs of contributors and conditions under which a certain amount can be withdrawn:

Account I constitutes 60 per cent of a member's savings for retirement in accordance to the primary objective of the scheme, to ensure that members have sufficient cash savings for retirement. Up to 20 per cent of the balance in Account I can be transferred for investment purposes. This is a new feature introduced in 1996 to allow contributors to invest under the Members' Saving Investment Scheme.

Account II (30 per cent) allows a member to withdraw savings once for buying or building a house. This withdrawal is limited to 20 per cent of the price of the house or 45 per cent of the savings but not exceeding RM20,000. Under this account, members will also be allowed to withdraw some money to finance the cost of their children's education.

Account III (10 per cent) is intended to help members to pay for critical illness expenses. This assistance, in the form of emergency medical expenses, allows 10 per cent of the contribution to be withdrawn. It is not limited to the member only, but extends to the member's spouse, children, parents and siblings.

From the introduction of the EPF until 1977, a lump sum payment was the mode of withdrawal upon retirement. In 1977, periodic payment withdrawal was introduced to allow members of retirement age to withdraw their savings periodically (once a month), until all savings were withdrawn. However, this method has not been popular (see for example *New Straits Times* 9 May 1999). Indeed, as of 31 December, 1999, only 176 members representing 0.24 per cent of overall members had chosen the monthly payment option (*The Edge* 6 November 2000). The EPF also provides two other methods of withdrawal. One is a part lump sum and part periodic payment (introduced in 1994), while the other (introduced in 1982) allows contributors to maintain the principal amount with the EPF, withdrawing only the annual dividends. In July 2000, the EPF introduced a further option, the annuity scheme, which aims to provide members with an even income stream throughout their retirement years. This annuity scheme received a mixed response and, indeed, following objections from the Malaysian Trade Union Congress, it was suspended in May 2001.

Coverage of the EPF

As of the end of December 1999, the total number of members was 9.54 million, comprising 4.78 million (50.1 per cent) active members, up from 3.99 million (or 51.4 per cent) active members in 1995 (Table 4.7), an increase of approximately 20 per cent.

TABLE 4.7

Malaysia: Number of Employees, Provident Fund (EPF) Members, 1995–99

Year	Total Number of Members (million)	Number of Active Members[a] (million)	Percentage of Active Members[a]	Total Labour Force (million)	Percentage of Active Members[a] to Labour Force
1995	7.76	3.99	51.4%	8.26	48.3%
1996	8.05	4.18	51.9%	8.64	48.4%
1997	8.27	4.31	52.1%	9.04	47.7%
1998	9.16	4.66	50.9%	8.88	52.5%
1999	9.54	4.78	50.1%	9.01	53.1%

[a] Active members are those who have at least one contribution in the last twelve months.
Source: Employees' Provident Fund, *Annual Report* (1999); Ministry of Finance, Malaysia (1998–2001).

The relevance of the EPF scheme as a source of financial support for Malaysia's current cohort of elderly population may not be significant, for three reasons. First, a large proportion of older persons in the present cohort are in the informal sector, in which contributions are not made mandatory. However, given the choice to make contributions towards their old age, most informal sector workers do not do so, for a variety of reasons. Workers in the informal sector, where official retirement often does not apply, usually work until they are unable to do so due to ill health. Secondly, there always remains the question of whether people will have enough in their EPF accounts to see them through their lives, if the EPF is the only source of income (Mehta 1997a). Rising costs associated with longer life expectancy and the effects of inflation will diminish the value of savings. Thirdly, the lump-sum nature of withdrawals tends to mean high exposure to improper management or investments that do not provide the security needed for old age.

The EPF has conducted several simulations to assess the extent to which the fund addresses the issue of adequacy (Kumar 1997). Based on the ILO Convention, 1952 no. 102, the minimum replacement rate is at least 40 per cent of the last drawn salary. Simulations conducted in 1995 on various categories of contributors show that the monthly annuity payment receivable for a period of 20 years for the manual, clerical and executive categories were, respectively, 58 per cent, 53 per cent and 40 per cent of the last salary drawn, indicating a sufficient replacement rate (Kumar 1997). However, due to leakages prior to retirement in the form of the withdrawals permissible under different circumstances, and also because the EPF is not inflation-indexed, to guarantee adequacy for life remains the main challenge for the scheme.

Health care

Many of the concerns and much of the panic over health and ageing populations relate to the burden that this can allegedly place on the health care system, especially associated with rising costs. In terms of health status, based on self-assessment, the majority of older persons felt that they were healthy, with a higher percentage stating this among urban elderly people (Chen et al. 1986; Chia 1996; Tan et al. 1999). A higher proportion of males than females rated their health as "very good" or "good" (Chen and Jones, 1989). Common health problems included eyesight problems (with women over 75 years being the worst affected) and evidence of cataracts, and difficulty in chewing with some needing dental prosthesis (Chen et al. 1986; Chen and Jones 1989; Tan et al. 1999). Eyesight problems were more prevalent among older persons than were hearing problems. According to Tan et al. (1999), about 40 per cent of older people indicted that they had specific health problems, with a higher percentage of women than men suffering from this. High blood pressure seemed the most common problem, again affecting more females than males. Rheumatism was a problem for women, but hardly seemed to affect males; likewise for joint problems (Chia 1996). Unsurprisingly, a higher proportion of the oldest-old were affected than were the younger-old.

On the whole, a high percentage of older persons could cope with all the activities of daily living (ADLs), as is shown in Table 4.8. A higher proportion of male oldest-old people (75 years of age and over) than females could do so (Chen et al. 1986). Similarly, in a separate study of a semi-rural district, it was found that 80 per cent of men between 65 and 74, and 64 per cent of men over 75, could manage all the ADLs whilst, among females, the percentages were 71 per cent and 68 per cent, respectively (Chia 1996). Again, ability to perform ADLs deteriorated with age. Among those who could not perform all the ADLs, the main difficulties encountered were walking and shopping. "Getting in and/or out of bed" was a problem only to the oldest-old group, more so for females than males. On the whole, men seemed to have better physical health than women, especially among the older age groups aged 70 years and over.

On a cognitive score, people aged 75 years and over performed worst in respect of *mental health* (Chen et al. 1986). Cognitive scores for elderly men were higher than that for women (Table 4.9). Both genders reported being worried/tense, having lost interest, feeling tired, being forgetful and paranoid. In the cognitive assessment, the proportion of elderly people who managed a normal score decreased with age, and women appeared to be more cognitively impaired than men. Controlling

TABLE 4.8

Malaysia: Number and Percentage per Age Group of Older Persons unable to Perform Activities of Daily Living (ADL)

Type of Activity	Male			Female			Total male and female
	60–74 Number (%)	75+ Number (%)	Total male Number (%)	60–74 Number (%)	75+ Number (%)	Total female Number (%)	Number (%)
Travel beyond walking distance	5 (1.0)	5 (5.0)	10 (2.0)	4 (1.0)	7 (7.0)	11 (2.0)	21 (2.0)
Go shopping	11 (3.0)	15 (6.0)	26 (5.0)	14 (3.0)	19 (19.0)	33 (6.0)	59 (6.0)
Handle own money	8 (2.0)	5 (5.0)	13 (3.0)	7 (2.0)	11 (11.0)	18 (4.0)	31 (3.0)
Eat	1 (0.3)	1 (1.0)	2 (0.4)	1 (0.0)	2 (2.0)	3 (0.6)	5 (0.5)
Dress self	1 (0.3)	5 (5.0)	6 (1.0)	0 (0.0)	2 (2.0)	2 (0.4)	8 (0.8)
Take care of appearance	1 (0.3)	3 (3.0)	4 (1.0)	0 (0.0)	2 (2.0)	2 (0.4)	6 (0.6)
Walk	2 (1.0)	1 (1.0)	3 (0.6)	1 (0.2)	4 (4.0)	5 (1.0)	8 (0.8)
Get in/out of bed	0 (0.0)	1 (1.0)	1 (0.2)	0 (0.0)	3 (3.0)	3 (0.6)	4 (0.4)
Take bath	1 (0.3)	4 (4.0)	5 (1.0)	0 (0.0)	3 (3.0)	3 (0.6)	8 (0.8)
Get to toilet on time	12 (3.0)	8 (9.0)	20 (4.0)	9 (2.0)	9 (9.0)	18 (4.0)	38 (4.0)
Sample size	**396**	**93**	**489**	**411**	**101**	**512**	**1001**

Source: Chen et al. (1986).

TABLE 4.9
Malaysia: Number and Percentage per Age Group of Older Persons Who Have Mental Health Problems

Type of Problems	Male			Female			Total male and female
	60–74 Number (%)	75+ Number (%)	Total male Number (%)	60–74 Number (%)	75+ Number (%)	Total female Number (%)	Number (%)
Sleep difficulties	110 (28)	36 (39)	146 (30)	150 (36)	40 (40)	190 (37)	336 (36)
Worried tense	59 (5)	18 (19)	77 (16)	115 (28)	32 (32)	147 (29)	224 (22)
Lost interest	108 (27)	39 (42)	147 (30)	119 (29)	41 (41)	160 (31)	307 (31)
Depressed	13 (3)	5 (5)	18 (4)	8 (2)	1 (1)	9 (2)	27 (3)
Feels tired	163 (41)	47 (51)	210 (43)	209 (51)	56 (55)	265 (55)	475 (47)
Forgetful	502 (52)	53 (57)	258 (53)	249 (61)	69 (69)	318 (62)	576 (58)
Hears things	6 (2)	3 (3)	9 (2)	6 (1)	5 (5)	11 (2)	20 (2)
Sees things	8 (2)	2 (2)	10 (2)	6 (1)	5 (5)	11 (2)	21 (2)
Paranoid	7 (2)	3 (3)	10 (2)	11 (3)	1 (1)	12 (2)	22 (2)
Sample size	396	93	489	411	101	512	1001

Source: Chen et al. (1986).

for the effects of age, cognitive scores were significantly correlated to ADLs, regardless of gender (Chia 1996). Cognitive function was related to other socio-economic variables, for example, those with inadequate income were more likely than the economically stable to report sleep difficulties, loss of enthusiasm in life and were more likely to have a cognitive score of less than 11 out of 14 (Chen et al.1986).

Social health includes, amongst other things, perception of environment, participation in activities and ways of life. Almost all older Malaysians, males and females, rated their home environment as fair, good or excellent, except for a small percentage who did not feel safe in their homes (Chen et al.1986). Tan et al. (1999) found that the majority of older people lived with their spouse or children, indicating that support is available to them, whether it be emotional, social or financial. Only a small percentage stated that they did not have anyone to provide care when they were ill, whereas the majority had someone to care for them. Older persons were still able to care for their grandchildren (Chen et al. 1986). Slightly more than half helped to make family decisions, with men playing a greater role than women.

Some 60 per cent of older persons indicated that they were interested in community activities, and a higher proportion of men than women (Tan et al. 1999). Malays appeared to be more interested than the non-Malays, and rural people were more interested than the urban dwellers. However, the percentage this actually involved was rather low. About one-quarter of older persons were members of social organizations, but the majority of these did not participate or participated only occasionally. Only 4 per cent reported that they belonged to some group, meeting or society for elderly or retired people (Chen et al. 1986). More participated in private functions such as family functions. Among both males and females, attendance declined with age, with the decline being more pronounced for women. There were no differences between rural and urban areas.

Slightly more than 40 per cent of elderly men and almost 20 per cent of women reported that they smoked (Chen et al. 1986).

One fifth of elderly men and only 3 per cent of women indicated that they smoked 15 or more cigarettes per day although many were light smokers.

Use of health services

On average, Malaysians visit the public and private primary care service sector about 2.3 times per year, but older persons made an average of 6 visits per year (Chia 1996). Government health services were the most popular choice for all age groups, regardless of gender. Chen et al. (1986) and Tan et al. (1999) found that fewer than 50 per cent of older persons surveyed reported having fallen ill and only a negligible percentage had been hospitalized. More females had been ill than males, across the age groups. About half of elderly respondents had taken prescribed medicines, with no age, sex or urban–rural differences. Some preferred to seek the help of traditional medication, either Malay or Chinese. Some just bought over-the-counter (OTC) medicine, which was related positively to feelings of ill health, with people who reported that they did not feel well being 10–15 per cent more likely to take OTC than those who reported that they felt healthy. There were no differences in the perceptions of need for more health aids in terms of age and sex, but rural residents were twice as likely as urban residents to express a need for more health services. This could be due to rural–urban differences in terms of accessibility and type of health facilities (quantity and quality).

Existing policies and programmes for health care

A review of existing policies and programmes is linked with a review of public support for health care in terms of total personnel available, public health facilities and coverage. Currently, there is a dearth of professional expertise, with only three geriatricians, three gerontologists and two psycho-geriatricians to care for the increasing number of elderly people (Table 4.10).

TABLE 4.10

Malaysia: Available Trained Health-Care Personnel for Older Persons

Category	Number
Geriatricians	3
Gerontologists	3
Psycho-geriatricians	2
Rehabilitation physicians	5
Physiotherapists	260
Occupational therapists	120
Speech therapists	14
Clinical psychologists	10

Source: First National Symposium on Gerontology 1995, data from The Family Health Division of the Ministry of Health.

An important development in the care for older persons has been the establishment of geriatric care in Malaysia. Since the mid-1990s, geriatric hospitals and rehabilitation centres have opened for services to older persons. For example, the Seremban Hospital (a public hospital) provides geriatric care, while the University Malaya Medical Center in Kuala Lumpur operates a geriatric unit. Only one private hospital in Malaysia caters specifically for older persons (located in Shah Alam in the state of Selangor). Another geriatric hospital has been granted approval during the Seventh Plan period with several other hospitals in the planning stage for geriatric service (Eighth Malaysia Plan 2001–2005). Of the total number of 33 hospitals approved during the Seventh Plan Period, 16 hospitals will provide geriatric service while one in the state of Selangor is designed to provide only rehabilitative and geriatric care (Eighth Malaysia Plan 2001–2005). In addition to services available in the public sector, several private hospitals have also set up geriatric service. Rehabilitative services such as physiotherapy and occupational therapy are available to older people as a support service, although this does not extend to rural areas. Thus, it can be seen that although the network of hospitals and clinics in the country provides medical and health care to all age groups, including older persons, progressive efforts are being made to provide care for older persons. As part of the caring society concept, for example, parents of civil servants are given free medical services in government hospitals and special counters are being created for older persons to receive medication.

Financing for health care

Since the cost of health care is a major concern for individuals, families and the Malaysian government, it is imperative to understand the financial resources that are available for health care. The significance of finance has been explicitly acknowledged in the Eighth Malaysia Plan 2001–2005 as one of the strategies for health sector development: "developing and instituting a healthcare financing scheme" (p. 491) although no details of the strategy are currently available. Several sources of financing can be distinguished: allocations from the government, out-of-pocket expenses reimbursed as a benefit provided by employers (private sector), and health insurance. Of these modes of financing, the most significant for older persons are allocation from the government and out-of-pocket expenses. Among employees in the public sector, retired government servants can continue to enjoy medical benefits at government clinics and hospitals. Medical insurance is a fairly recent development in Malaysia and it is not yet a significant source of financing; moreover, it appeals more to urban people, who are the only ones who can afford to purchase such insurance. Allocations from the government have been a feature of the annual government budget and form an important source of health care provision.

A national survey has been conducted on household health expenditure (although the data are not yet publicly available), but such a lack of information on health expenditure is not unique to Malaysia and has been widely reported in many developing countries. In general, the main means of payment for health care in Malaysia is people's own out-of-pocket payments, whilst the least popular means of payment is insurance (Table 4.11). The importance of out-of-pocket payments increases with age and formed 75 per cent of payments among those aged 60 and above — whereas, unsurprisingly, insurance did not feature at all for this age group.

TABLE 4.11
Malaysia: Sources of Payment for Health Care, 1996 (percentages)

Characteristics	Self (Out-of-Pocket)	Free	Employer	Insurance	Donation	Other Sources	Self, and Employer Insurance	Self and Employer	Other Combinations
Location									
Urban	62.2	3.1	18.7	0.1	0.0	5.3	5.0	2.9	2.6
Rural	66.4	5.3	11.7	0.1	0.0	7.0	3.6	1.6	4.1
Age Group									
0–14	67.7	5.2	7.7	0.1	0.0	10.0	4.1	1.2	3.8
15–59	60.6	3.3	22.2	0.1	0.0	3.3	4.4	3.2	2.8
60+	75.1	4.4	3.9	0.0	0.1	6.8	5.6	0.7	3.1

Source: National Health and Morbidity Survey (1996).

The 1995 Health Care Programme for the Elderly

This programme, introduced in 1995, aimed to improve and maintain the health and functional ability of older persons, with the ultimate objective of promoting quality of life as well as forging productive ageing among older persons. Specific objectives included:

1. To improve the health of older persons to enable them to lead and enjoy full and active lives through promotive and preventive health care
2. To establish specialist geriatric services at the regional and state levels by 2000
3. To develop a comprehensive plan of action on training and research needs in the care of older persons
4. To provide quality health care for older persons using community-based approaches to enable them to live as independently as possible within the community.

Various primary and secondary components of health care have been identified, and strategies formulated, to achieve the objectives of the programme, which include the following:

Promotive and preventive health care.   This involves the dissemination of information regarding pathologies and disabilities related to age. Regular screening programmes will be conducted to check for conditions such as visual and hearing impairment, coronary artery diseases, breast cancer and oral cancer. Pre-retirement courses related to health, financial security, volunteerism and use of leisure time are also planned for people nearing this age of transition.

Medical and rehabilitative care.   This aims to strengthen care for older persons at primary, secondary and tertiary levels. One strategy is to provide holistic specialized medical, psychological, social and rehabilitative geriatric services in selected state and district hospitals using a multi-disciplinary team approach. From the regulatory perspective, the Private Hospitals Act, 1971 and Private Hospital Regulations, 1973, will be enforced to ensure quality care for older persons.

Training and research. These are needed to formulate and strengthen the existing curricula on care of older persons for basic, post-basic and continuing medical education. Training is planned in specialist areas relating to the health care of older persons according to projected manpower needs. In addition, a focal point for coordinating research activities in the medical and social aspects of caring for older persons will be established to ensure a coordinated approach towards researching the issues affecting this age group.

Programme planning, monitoring, coordination and evaluation. As routine data collection generally does not meet the information requirements, actions should be directed to correct data gaps. An action plan is in place for proper data collection in hospitals and health centres in order to obtain more accurate information about older persons. Strategies include establishing a special unit on health care for the elderly in the Family Health Development Division of the Ministry of Health.

Since the initiation of this programme, some progress has been made, with some examples of activities being:

1. A National Plan of Action on Community Mental Health programme was established in 1997 and some pilot projects have been carried out in health clinics in Johor, Malacca, Negeri Sembilan, Kedah and Sabah. Training was conducted to upgrade the knowledge and skills of health personnel. The National Mental Health Policy was approved in 1998 and 58 health clinics have been identified to implement the programme. Activities have included talks, forums and exhibitions on mental health, follow-up for stable mental cases, early detection of mental disorders, group therapy, home visits, counselling, rehabilitation, screening, setting up of day-care centres at health clinics, training for health personnel and the development and distribution of educational materials on aspects of mental health.
2. A healthy lifestyle campaign aimed at preventing and controlling chronic diseases such as diabetes mellitus and cardiovascular disease.

3. Rehabilitative services such as physiotherapy and occupational therapy are provided to older people as a supportive service to medical care or in-patient care in hospitals, although these services are not available in the rural areas.

4. Health centre or community-based activities planned include home visits; health screening for high-risk groups; referral to geriatricians; counselling on exercise, nutrition, diabetics and social support needs; home mobility and rehabilitative facilities; special care management, such as for incontinence; day-care nursing; and community education on issues associated with the health of older persons.

5. Hospital-based activities, including acute medical care, long-term care, psycho-geriatric care, therapy and patient education, were initiated.

6. Plans for 1997–2000 include the development of two main services — hospital services and health centres or community health services — to be delivered mainly by the Department of Social Welfare, NGOs, private and voluntary organizations.

In addition to the overall challenge of providing more specialized health care for older persons, it is important to note the uneven availability of health care in urban and rural areas, as the expertise and facilities are generally lacking in the latter. Health and health-related services that are available to older persons in the urban areas through private organizations are generally not available to rural elderly people, as their purchasing power is low. Hence, in the rural areas, elderly people are seen as out-patients in health centres, with referrals made to hospitals for more serious cases. This geographical divide in health care for older persons needs to be addressed and eliminated, but income differentials between the wealthy and the poor remains an obstacle to achieving accessibility and coverage for all. Exactly how quality health care can be made more egalitarian for older Malaysians remains a great challenge.

Social services and community care

In caring for elderly people, both the family and the community have long been perceived as of primary importance (Chow 1992). In the case of most developing countries such as Malaysia, where competing needs are varied and other issues are sometimes regarded as more urgent than the seemingly less important ones relating to older persons, family and community care seem to be the most viable alternative to the welfare state approach. In addition, the deeply rooted Asian culture that stresses the importance of filial piety has in the past dictated that the family should provide care and security for the elderly. However, as discussed in Chapter 1, in Malaysia and many other countries in the region, the erosion of the extended family system, a decrease in the number of available female members due to the increase in female labour force participation, and smaller family sizes have combined to place strain on the family as the primary care giver. This development has created something of a gap that has motivated the development of institutional care. However, institutional care is often only accessible to those who can afford it (in the case of private nursing homes) and is mostly available only in the urban areas. Therefore, the argument for older persons to remain within the community has heralded the emergence of community care for older persons in Malaysia's fast industrializing society. Admission to public old persons' homes under the Department of Social Welfare is a last resort, and is provided only to elderly people who have no heirs and no shelter, or to those who are destitute. However, between those who have the means to purchase services and those who have very limited financial resources, there exists a large group who cannot be classified into either of these two extremes.

Social welfare services

Services to older persons are divided into two broad types under the Social Welfare Department: external services, and institutional services, aimed at providing services to poor older persons. The types of aid given are financial aid and material assistance, which includes items such as spectacles. Institutional care refers to shelter provided in old people's homes (*Rumah Seri Kenangan*) of which there are 11 (2 in East Malaysia) administered by the federal government. These homes offer accommodation, counselling and guidance, occupational rehabilitation, devotional facilities, recreational activities and medical treatment.

In the rural areas, assistance is given to elderly people for building new huts or to repair their existing ones, so that they can continue to stay within the community instead of having to be institutionalized. There are some 30 huts, housing about 300 residents, under the Central Welfare Council of Malaysia (MPKSM).

In addition to residential homes, the government allocated financial aid to more than 7 million elderly people, between 1995 to 1999 (Table 4.12). A total of RM11 million (US$3 million) was allocated to older persons in 1999, as well as offering aid in terms of spectacles. However, over the period 1995 to 1999, the number of aid recipients declined by 66 per cent from 758 to 255.

TABLE 4.12
Malaysia: Expenditure and Number of Older Persons Receiving Government-Allocation Financial Aid, 1995–99

Year	Number of Elderly Aid Recipients	Expenditure	Number of Elderly Aid Recipients for Spectacles	Expenditure (RM)
1995	10,049	8,697,630	758	17,604
1996	10,429	8,448,130	769	52,115
1997	11,793	7,898,624	591	37,309
1998	11,143	7,149,000	406	24,095
1999	13,903	11,040,444	255	20,922

Source: Department of Social Welfare, Malaysia (1995–99).

Long-term care

Perhaps the most obvious government effort in the provision of formal long-term care (LTC) has been the setting up of homes for the chronically ill. At present there are two centres — one in Kuala Kubu Baru, Selangor and the other in Dungun, Terengganu — with a total capacity of about 150, providing care, treatment and protection to chronically-ill older persons aged 60 years and above. The range of services and facilities also includes medical treatment, guidance and counselling, physiotherapy, devotional guidance, religious activities and recreational activities. Usually, residents remain for the rest of their lives in these homes.

In terms of medical services for the purpose of LTC, public hospitals, for example, the Seremban General Hospital, provide services such as home nursing, home visits by doctors, follow-up geriatric clinics, assessment and training for domestic maids to ensure that they are able to care for older persons, rehabilitation and visits to homes for the aged. They also run clinics and health assessments for residents.

Community care

To what extent community care is practiced in Malaysia? To outline the development of community care in Malaysia, "Williams' Ring" (Figures 4.1 and 4.2) can serve as a guide to the types of services possibly required by older persons, compared with the types of services available in Malaysia. As discussed above, while the family still remains the main source of care today, and is expected to do so in the future, community-based activities can help to alleviate the pressures on the family of providing care on a long-term basis. In Figure 4.1, the outermost ring refers to people's ability to perform social activities; the middle ring represents activities related to household chores; and the innermost ring represents the ability to perform self-care. As the process of ageing progresses, functional ability may be expected to decline, as depicted by the inward movement of the rings, with a decline in the

FIGURE 4.1

Malaysia: A Model of Social Performance Levels Among Older Persons

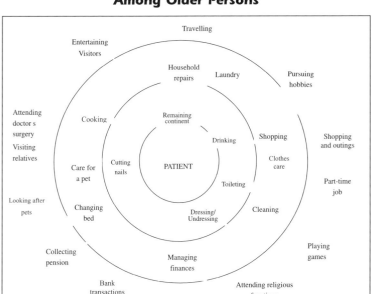

Source: After Williams (1996).

ability to perform activities, ranging from social activities to household chores and, finally, to personal care. At each stage of the potential decline, different kinds of assistance are required.

Perhaps the major issue that confronts Malaysia is the scale and scope of these services rather than the service per se, as most of the services (as marked in italic and bold in Figure 4.2) are now available, although not always formally or extensively. For example, for respite care, Malaysia has not yet reached a stage where the service is provided on an organized basis; rather, it is available informally, provided by those who are related or known to the family. Although the Central Welfare Council of Malaysia (MPKSM) has plans to set up respite care in the future, details of the plan are not currently available.

FIGURE 4.2

Malaysia: A Model of Services Available to Older Persons

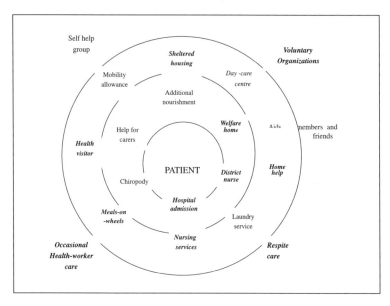

Self help group
Voluntary Organizations
Mobility allowance
Sheltered housing
Day -care centre
Additional nourishment
Welfare home
Aids
members and friends
Health visitor
Help for carers
Chiropody
PATIENT
District nurse
Home help
Meals-on -wheels
Hospital admission
Laundry service
Occasional Health-worker care
Nursing services
Respite care

Services (in italics and bold) available in Malaysia.
Respite care refers to a non-organized form of care — that provided by family members and friends.
Source: After Williams (1996).

Domiciliary care

Domiciliary care is one of the most common community-based services for older people and can include basic care (help with daily living, mobility and self care), home nursing and home visiting (Tinker 1996). In the UK, for example, the home-help service has been noted as the most important feature of domiciliary support. In Malaysia, home-help services and home visiting are currently rather limited, while home nursing services are provided by the public and private sectors, as well as by voluntary bodies (Awang 1992). Such nursing is not specifically for older persons, but is available to all who are eligible and can afford to pay (except for services sponsored by the government, such as midwifery and child care in the rural areas).

TABLE 4.13
Malaysia: Recipients of Home-Help Service Provided by the MPKSM, 2000

Age Group	Male				Female				Total
	Malay	Chinese	Indian	Others	Malay	Chinese	Indian	Others	
60–65	6	28	1	—	30	18	1	—	84
66–70	15	16	7	2	41	2	1	—	84
70 above	28	82	7	3	83	50	2	4	259
Not known	14	11	7	4	18	8	—	2	64
Total	63	137	22	9	172	78	4	6	491

Source: MPKSM, Program Report, (2000).

Under the Central Welfare Council of Malaysia (MPKSM, or Majlis Pusat Kabajikan Senanjung Malaysia), a scheme known as "the home help service" is offered to older persons, and its services include home visits, hospital visits, occupational therapy, simple medical tests and counselling in an out-reach programme. In 1990, a total of 66 caregivers offered services to 491 elderly people, with those aged 70 years and above forming the largest group (Table 4.13). In East Malaysia, the home help service was introduced in 2000; in Sabah, there were 159 registered elderly clients and 275 home visits were made (MPKSM, various records).

The Golden age Foundation (*Usiamas*), dating from 1991, is another NGO also involved in domiciliary care, providing nursing care and home visits to older persons, in particular those newly discharged from hospital. It operates in Melaka, a southern state in Peninsular Malaysia and, for home nursing, referrals are mainly from the Melaka General Hospital, although a small number are from the Social Welfare Department. In addition, occasional social visits are made to older persons to lesson their feelings of loneliness. Day-centre services, training for caregivers and a resource centre for the ageing are also provided by the Golden age Foundation. To date, the home nursing service has benefited an average of over 300 older persons annually, with the figures for the use of nursing services and home visits both on the increase.

Day-care centres

Day-care centres are different from the day centres operated by MPKSM. Day centres offer a place for social interaction for independent older persons, whereas day-care centres provide care for older people who are not capable of performing some of the ADL. Day-care centres are premises in which four or more people receive for care for a continuous period exceeding three hours and for at least three days a week, whether for reward or otherwise. However, day-care centres are to be distinguished from residential care centres that provide care to elderly people who are residents in them. Currently, the MPKSM is in the initial stages of planning and building day-care centres for older persons; according to its chief executive, a total of 19 centres have been planned for the period 2000–02. The completion of these day care centres is hoped to greatly improve facilities for LTC.

Involvement of other non-governmental organizations in community care

It has been government policy in Malaysia to assist and encourage voluntary bodies to provide care for older persons. Accordingly, the government provides assistance in the form of grants to voluntary organizations to provide community services to older persons. The role of the National Council of Senior Citizens Organizations Malaysia (NACSCOM) may be highlighted here. Founded in 1990, it is a voluntary non-governmental, non-sectarian and non-profit federation of senior citizens' organizations in Malaysia, and currently comprises 23 senior citizens associations, and a total membership of more than 5,000.

The NACSCOM Advisory Council was formed in 1995 to implement programmes to foster better intergenerational understanding and interaction. A five-year plan of action was drawn up based on the framework of the National Policy for the Elderly, with expertise assistance from the United Nations Economic and Social Commission for Asia–Pacific (ESCAP). This plan of action has called for initiation and implementation in several areas of needs, such as income security, housing and legal affairs, education and training, health and medical services, sports and recreation, social services and welfare, information and publicity and fundraising. In terms of education and training, NACSCOM aims to organize educational courses or programmes to upgrade the skills of senior citizens or to assist them to acquire new skills which will help them to gain employment, should they desire to do so. NACSCOM also organizes seminars; forums on ageing issues, health, leisure and recreational activities; and training courses for volunteers for community out-reach programmes. In terms of health and medical services, NACSCOM is urging the authorities to plan and provide comprehensive health care facilities and services for older persons, and advocates employment of more geriatricians, specialized nurses and health workers for aged care. The plan of action also aims to initiate and support home nursing and convalescent day-care centres to allow sick older persons to remain in their own homes with their family for as long as possible, in line with the concept of a caring society promoted by the government.

Institutional care

In Malaysia, institutional care is delivered by three parties: the government in the provision of residential homes and LTC (as discussed above, under social welfare services); the private sector, which is motivated by profit and for which the ability to pay applies; and non-government organizations, which respond to the needs of older persons as well as to the encouragement of the government.

Nursing homes: private sector involvement

Nursing homes established in major urban areas reflect market forces, and demand is underpinned by the ability to purchase. The types of care nursing homes provide differ from home to home, but the basic facilities remain largely the same. Nursing homes run by private organizations are monitored by the Ministry of Health or the Social Welfare Department, and the first private nursing home was established in 1983. By 2001, it was estimated that there were about 40 to 50 moderate-sized nursing homes of about 40 beds or more in Malaysia, concentrated mainly in the Klang Valley and Penang, but there were hundreds more smaller homes in operation, usually with fewer than 10 beds, located in bungalows and other private residences (*The Edge*, 19 February 2001). These nursing homes offer 24-hour nursing care for people with different needs, including elderly and disabled people. Nursing homes could be regarded as formal facilities for long-term care (Cheah 1995) but the quality of care they provide is inconsistent (*The Edge*, 19 February 2001).

Of the hundreds of nursing homes estimated to be in operation throughout Malaysia, only 188 are licensed by the Social Welfare Department as qualified care centres. Of these, only 29 are nursing homes for older persons, accommodating 1,046 residents. Seven of these homes are run by NGOs and the remainder are private businesses owned by individuals. In 2001, the Social Welfare Department was processing another 45 applications from individuals and 20 from NGOs for licences to run elderly care centres (*The Edge*, 19 February 2001).

Non-government organizations in institutional care

Apart from the shelter provided by the government and private organizations, there are other residential homes known as *Rumah Sejahtera* (residential homes), administered by the Central Welfare Council of Malaysia (MPKSM), a non-government organization. These homes come under the supervision of the Department of Social Welfare, which disburses grants on a regular basis. Services available in *Rumah Sejahtera* under the MPKSM are similar to those provided by residential homes operated by the Social Welfare Department, under the Ministry of National Unity and Social Development. MPKSM records indicate that in 2001 there were about 115 such residential homes and huts in Peninsular Malaysia, housing 917 residents. These homes mostly cater for people without major functional disabilities. In reality, however, *Rumah Sejatera* can be considered as LTC facilities for residents whose health status deteriorates during their stay but who are reluctant to be relocated. Faced with such a situation, the MPKSM usually enlists some community help to provide care and assistance with ADL. In addition to the non-medical care services, district health centres provide regular medical care to residents.

Implications of ageing in Malaysia

As in many countries of the region, economic development, medical advancements, accessibility to medical and social care and knowledge of nutrition have put more years into life, while the present and future challenges are recognized to be to put quality into these added years. For Malaysia, coping with population ageing can be a great challenge, as there are many competing issues that appear to deserve more urgent attention than that of improving the well-being of older persons. Indeed, the Eighth Malaysia Plan 2001–2005 does not have a separate chapter on the elderly, hinting that ageing has yet to become a national priority. Although Malaysia still has time on its side, ageing must attain the priority it deserves due to its multiple and complex social and economic implications.

Social security

In Malaysia, social security covers only employees in the formal sector. The Labour Force Survey Report of 1998 indicated that the percentage of total employed persons covered by the two schemes discussed earlier, the Pensions and Employees Provident Fund (EPF), was 61.8 per cent, leaving the remaining 38.2 per cent without a known source of coverage. Of the 2.29 million self-employed people, only 23,307 had registered with EPF in 1998 (Kumar 1999). As this is on a voluntary contribution basis, the take-up rate largely depends on the individual. Two major obstacles that need to be overcome when introducing social security to the informal sector are to expand coverage to the majority in the informal sector, in particular those with seasonal incomes such as farmers and fishermen, and to monitor compliance among contributors. Another important issue in income security for old age is adequacy. The EPF is not inflation-indexed, and ensuring adequacy remains a great challenge. The lump-sum nature of withdrawal, which remains popular to date, poses another challenge. A concern is how best to invest/save/ utilize savings if funds are to last one's full life. In an attempt to achieve this, the government has introduced an annuity scheme for EPF members, but its success will only be apparent in the future.

Health and health financing

In Malaysia, a National Health for the Elderly Council was established under the Ministry of Health in 1997, and acts as the main body for monitoring policies pertaining to the health of older persons. The Family Health Development Division of the Public Health Department of the Ministry of Health serves as the secretariat of the Council. In the Plan of Action for Health of the Elderly enshrined in the National Policy for the Elderly, health facilities for optimum care involve:

- strengthening coordination and collaboration between government and non-government agencies, including the private sector in providing health services
- planning and providing promotive, curative and rehabilitative services
- providing the appropriate physical, personnel and financial facilities for the programme
- encouraging community involvement in the care and rehabilitation of older persons, and
- encouraging training and research.

Although there exists a plan of action on health care for older persons, the delivery of care remains integrated into the health care provisions of the broader system, through primary care and secondary and tertiary services. Special hospitals for older persons are limited, although there exists positive development toward the provision of specific health care, as in geriatric care, for older persons, by both the public and private sectors, and the intention is to introduce geriatric care in all district hospitals by year 2020. However, achieving this target will be difficult, considering the lack of expertise in geriatrics. In addition, as elsewhere, health financing remains a great challenge with rising needs and costs relating to health care. Although the *Eighth Malaysia Plan 2001–2005* proposes a strategy for a health care financing scheme, it is still too early to speculate on its outcome. At present, out-of-pocket payments form the main mode of financing, especially for the oldest-old age group.

Community care

It is clear that community care needs to be further developed both in scale and scope. The emerging preference for nuclear families and the increasing participation of females in the formal sector implies that family care has to be supplemented with other forms of care, whether for reward or otherwise, to allow the family to continue to provide care to older persons. More fiscal incentives may have to be put in place to encourage the community to be involved in community care but, apart from such measures, increased allocations may have to be channeled as seed money for the development of community care projects. To overcome the increasing costs of labour and to encourage productive ageing, voluntarism among able-bodied older persons will also be beneficial for community care.

Conclusion and future directions

The National Policy for the Elderly 1995 and the National Health for the Elderly Council established in 1997 represent milestones in Malaysia in providing care and services to older persons. The two ministries responsible for services for older persons are the Ministry of National Unity and Social Development, through the Department of Welfare Services, and the Ministry of Health. The National Policy provides the broad framework for the development of care and services to older persons. Equally important is the delivery mechanism that must take account of geographical divides, the uneven distribution of facilities between urban and rural areas, and the varying needs of differing groups — such as women, who may be particularly vulnerable, and the oldest-old, who have more needs compared to the young-old, who are likely to be more independent.

Notable progress has been made over recent years in the development of care for older persons and Malaysia has been classified, with the Republic of Korea and Guam, as a country that has made recent initiatives in the development of health services (World Health Organization 1998). It is hoped that Malaysia will soon become a country that has an established system of care for older persons, not only in terms of health, but also in other areas that affect their overall quality of life.

In attempting to predict the future direction of policy and provision for older persons in Malaysia, one may begin with the sources or determinants of and improvements to the quality of life of older persons. While searching for innovative ways to provide care for older persons, the potential of elderly people themselves in development should not be ignored. Broad suggestions for improvements include the following:

Census-type information.   This needs to be gathered to facilitate the formulation and implementation of policies and programmes. It is hoped that the research sub-committee of the Action Plan for the National Policy on the Elderly will be able to fill the data gaps.

Government intervention at the macro level.   Potential loss of productivity and higher social costs may be associated with demographic ageing, but many interventions can mitigate such costs (Joaquin-Yasay 1996). These include adjustments in retirement age, training and effective employment of older women, better education and training for young people and appropriate policies for regulating migration and temporary foreign labour. Some of these interventions already exist in Malaysia. Indeed, a new retirement age has recently been announced, now 56 years instead of the 55 years previously. Challenges remain for elderly women, who are generally less educated, less financially independent and may be exposed to greater health risks than men. Interim measures can be taken to provide protection to this vulnerable group, as the profile of future cohorts of elderly women is likely to be very different and less dependent than the present cohort.

Social security.   Taking into account the economic structure and development in Malaysia, a single approach to social security, whether by defined benefits or defined contributions, is unlikely to be feasible as it will not provide coverage to all sectors of the population. A combination of approaches is essential, as this can enhance stability. The prevention of leakages of funds before retirement should be minimized, as opposed to the present system in which numerous withdrawals are permitted.

Access to comprehensive health care.   Health promotion and preventive care should be emphasized further and the uneven accessibility of health care services in the urban and rural areas needs urgent attention.

Training of personnel.   This is particularly important in the health sector if better care is to reach a larger number of elderly people. There are various types of training programmes available: post-basic geriatric nursing, in-service training for primary health care staff and in-service training for carers, who are medical assistants and nurses. It is important to introduce geriatric medicine and other gerontology-related disciplines in the training of medical and allied personnel.

Health care financing.   It is recognized that the cost of health care can be a major barrier to the accessibility and use of care. As such, ensuring an adequate system of health financing is a major policy issue, and a national approach to development of policies for health financing, health insurance and medical, pharmaceutical and health care services payment is essential (World Health Organization 1998). On whatever approach or approaches the national policy on health care financing is modelled, the underlying principle should be that no-one is denied basic health care.

Education and retraining for older persons.   Developing programmes to retrain older persons can help to realize the principles of independence, participation and self-fulfillment which, for the two decades since the Vienna World Assembly on Ageing, have been widely held in many countries and were reaffirmed at the 2002 Madrid World Assembly. Education to prepare older persons for the challenges of ageing can be introduced in the form of pre-retirement courses, whilst retraining can help to promote productive ageing.

Innovative employment opportunities for older persons.   These can help to promote productivity among older persons. Although protecting the employment and welfare of older citizens is important, generating work opportunities for the young is often equally, if not more, important in industrializing countries such as Malaysia. A flexible wage structure may allow older people to continue working, after the mandatory retirement age. Alternatively, older persons can be redeployed to areas of work that require, for example, less physical strength or abilities. Intergenerational strategies can be developed in which younger-old persons can begin to offer their services to the oldest-old group or to young children, whether for reward or otherwise, so that they can "free" working-age adults to concentrate on their jobs. In this way, whilst their contribution is indirect, it can help to instil a sense of worth and fulfilment among older persons, although mobilizing some older persons can pose a challenge.

Housing, environmental and town planning.   In anticipating the growth of an ageing population, planning for townships should take into account the facilities and environmental needs of older persons. In line with policy for older persons to remain in the community, infrastructure enabling the mobility of older persons is important and should be incorporated thoroughly into town planning.

Avoidance of the duplication of services.   Optimizing the utilization of scarce resources is crucial, while leaving gaps in the provision of services can be a barrier to a better quality of life for older persons. In order to avoid the duplication or under-delivery of services, a new ministry may be necessary to formulate or coordinate policies that will optimize the provision of care and protection to older persons, instead of sub-optimizing from the fragmentation and malcoordination of different functions and activities.

5

National Policies on Ageing and Long-term Care in Singapore
A Case of Cautious Wisdom?

Kalyani K. Mehta

Introduction

In the context of the Asia–Pacific region, Singapore represents a unique case of a rapidly ageing, geographically small nation characterized by its multi-ethnic and multi-lingual population. According to the 2000 Population Census, there were about four million people in Singapore, of whom 3.263 million were citizens or permanent residents (Government of Singapore Census of Population, 2000), living in the city–state's total area of about 660 square kilometres. The three major ethnic groups are the Chinese, Malays and Indians comprising, respectively, 79 per cent, 14 per cent and 6 per cent of the total population. The remaining 1 per cent consists of smaller groups such as Japanese, Eurasians and others. The four official languages in Singapore are English, Mandarin, Malay and Tamil.

While it is well-known that Singapore has one of the fastest ageing populations in the Asia–Pacific region, the speed of the demographic ageing process has been less emphasized. What developed countries experienced over a period of 80 to 100 or more years is being experienced in less than half the time in a number of countries such as Japan, Hong Kong and Singapore (Mehta 1999; ESCAP 1996a; Phillips 2000b). Figure 5.1 provides a graphic illustration of the rapidity of the demographic ageing process in Singapore. Table 5.1 summarizes Singapore's demographic projections to 2030.

FIGURE 5.1

Singapore: Persons Aged 65 and Above as a Percentage of the Total Population[a]

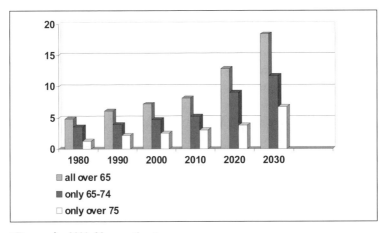

[a] Figures for 2000–30 are estimates.
Source: Inter-Ministerial Committee on Health Care for the Elderly (1999).

TABLE 5.1

Singapore: Number and Proportion of Older Persons[a]

	1999	2000	2020	2030
No. aged 65+ (in thousands)	235	312	529	796
Proportion aged 65 +*	7.3	8.4	13.1	18.9
Median age (years)	33.4	36.9	39.3	41.2
Dependency ratio (DR)	42.0	38.7	44.9	56.4
DR (Young) 0–14 years	31.7	27.1	25.9	26.9
DR (Old) 65+ years	10.4	11.6	19.0	29.5

[a] Figures for 2000–30 are estimates.
Source: Inter-Ministerial Committee on the Ageing Population (1999).

The development of policies on ageing

In the early 1980s, the Singapore Government began to recognise the likely impact an ageing population would have on society. In June 1982, a thirteen-member committee, The Committee on the Problems of the Aged, was appointed and it marked the beginning of the government's thrust to implement counter-measures in anticipation of the attendant problems of a demographically ageing population. The committee commissioned the first National Survey of Senior Citizens in 1983, the results of which were published in the *Report of the Committee on the Problems of the Aged* in 1984.

In tandem with the government's approach and philosophy of foresight and visionary planning, in 1984 an Inter-Ministerial Population Committee was set up. In 1988, the National Advisory Council on the Aged was formed to undertake a comprehensive review of the status of ageing in Singapore. One of the key recommendations proposed by the Advisory Council was that a National Council on Ageing should be set up with the character and authority of a statutory board to plan and coordinate policies and programmes for older persons effectively. Other proposals included raising the retirement age from 55 to 60, as continued employment provides a sense of worth, dignity and financial independence to older persons; adjusting the seniority-based wage system so that more older people will be employed; expanding and strengthening public education programmes for older persons and ageing, so that an appropriate attitude towards older persons could be inculcated; making land available for voluntary organizations to set up homes for older persons; lengthening the lease terms for homes; studying the feasibility of providing health and medical services for frail older people living in their own homes; and increasing the dependency tax rebate for families who look after older people. Among the many recommendations implemented was the establishment of a National Council on Family and Aged (NACFA), located at the Ministry of Community Development. Indeed,

> Within the period of about five decades, a shift has occurred in the philosophy regarding care for the elderly.

> In contrast to the wholly welfare-oriented approach of the 1940–60s, there has been evidence of a more balanced developmental-cum-welfare oriented approach from the 1970s to the present. (Mehta 1997*b*, p. 33)

To meet further challenges of population ageing, the 1990s saw the development of two milestone policies that were implemented to deal with anticipated problems related to the social and health care of older persons. Various community groups and the Parliamentary Select Committee introduced a significant legislation called the Maintenance of Parents Act in 1995, after many deliberations. There was public endorsement for the policy to impose a legal obligation on children to maintain their parents. Such a social policy deals with prevention and problems related to the neglect of elderly parents. In most urban societies, family breakdown is becoming a critical social problem and this will have consequences on quality of care and support for the elderly. In 1996, amendments to the Women's Charter provided channels for elderly parents to exercise legal action if they were victims of physical, mental or psychological abuse. Another enlightened policy covering medical care of terminally-ill people was put in place in 1996. More specifically, under the Advanced Medical Directive Act, persons medically certified brain dead can now under their earlier directives be relieved of medical life support. Such a progressive and futuristic policy has the potential to reduce unnecessary suffering to both the terminally-ill older persons and their families.

A national policy on ageing in Singapore has thus taken shape after a number of successive policy reviews, and two characteristics may be noted in the policy formulation process. First, the various committees have the benefit of representation from various sectors. This has the advantage of receiving diverse inputs and making implementable decisions. Historically, cross-sectoral representation has worked well in the local context and it is the standard feature in the Singapore Government's problem-solving approach. Second, the committees were given much publicity and public awareness of the issues was heightened especially when controversial recommendations were made. The enhanced discussion on policy changes by the public sees an increasing emphasis on the social care of older persons in Singapore. Public input thus became an important consideration in the committees' deliberations (Mehta and Vasoo 2000).

To summarize, five high-level committees have been appointed since 1982 to review the various issues and problems that are anticipated as an outcome of a rapidly ageing population (Vasoo et al. 2000). The most recent Inter-Ministerial Committee on the Ageing Population, formed in 1998, has considered many of the earlier recommendations of various committees on ageing matters. It has proposed a more coordinated and comprehensive plan to deal with the challenging issues of Singapore's ageing population in the twenty-first century.

In terms of funding policies for services for the elderly (as well as those for the general population), the state applies the "co-payment" principle as far as possible. The individual consumer and his/her family is expected to pay a portion of the charges while the government subsidizes the rest. This applies to the Medisave scheme, a compulsory medical savings scheme under the rubric of the Central Provident Fund (CPF), the Singaporean social security system. An individual may use his or her Medisave for his own or his parent's hospitalization expenses (including expenses incurred at a hospice). A sliding scale of charges is imposed, based on household income for community-based services such as home nursing, day-care and rehabilitation services. Recipients of Public Assistance, a financial scheme targeted towards destitute, frail or disabled elderly people and disbursed by the Ministry of Community Development and Sports (MCDS) are entitled to free medical services at the government polyclinics. All Singaporeans above 60 are entitled to a subsidy of 75 per cent of the fees charged at polyclinics.

A new strategy, implemented in September 2002, is a special insurance scheme, Eldershield, that provides coverage for disability, especially in old age (see p. 163). Such a scheme is warranted in view of the lengthening life expectancy of Singaporeans. The expectation of life at birth (ELB) in 1990 was 72 years for males and 78 for females, whereas in by 2050, it is likely to rise to 78 years for males and 82 for females (Shantakumar

1994). The reality is an even higher ELB. The rationale behind this type of scheme is that in the productive years, one should be able to put aside some savings for old age disability.

At present, the lead government ministry in charge of issues of ageing is the Ministry of Community Development and Sports (MCDS). However, it works closely with the other relevant ministries such as the Ministries of Health, Manpower, and Communications. The composition of the Inter-Ministerial Committee on Ageing Population reflects this policy of coordinating efforts in policy-making and decision-making. The twenty-one member committee, chaired by the minister for communications, with the minister of community development and sports and the minister for health and environment as deputy chairmen, comprises high-level representatives from the Ministries of Communications, Manpower, and Trade and Industry. Statutory bodies represented include the National Council of Social Service, the Singapore National Employers' Federation, and the People's Association. Civic organizations whose opinions are included are the Singapore Action Group of Elders (SAGE), the Tsao Foundation, and the Gerontological Society of Singapore. Whilst in the past a "top down" method of policy formulation was practised, a trend towards involving non-governmental organizations (NGOs) is slowly evolving.

Principal features of the national policies on ageing

> We want Singaporeans to age with dignity and to remain actively involved in society. We want them to be actively engaged in family and community life. And, in line with the Singapore 21 vision, we must maintain a strong sense of cohesion between the generations. Singapore should be the best home for all ages. (Inter-Ministerial Committee on the Ageing Population 1999, p. 13.).

This statement by Mr Goh Chok Tong, the prime minister, illustrates the main philosophy of the government with regard to issues of ageing. Singapore's government has clearly stated its stand that the "family is still the best approach — it provides the elderly with the warmth and companionship of family members and a level of emotional support that cannot be found elsewhere" (Minister of Health, Mr Yeo Chow Tong's keynote address at the Conference on Choices in Financing Health Care and Old Age Security 1997).

The present paradigm of care for the elderly in Singapore is a partnership between the government, the community and the family (Mehta 2000). In tandem with the "Many Helping Hands" policy of the MCDS, the community and the government are expected to lend a hand to ageing families in order to reduce the stress of taking care of older members. This policy emphasizes that the government expects to work hand-in-hand with civic bodies such as voluntary welfare organizations (VWOs), religious institutions, ethnic-based organizations and secular bodies such as clan associations. The support given to these organizations is in the form of funding, land leased at special rates, training of staff and guidance in programme planning. The Elderly Development Division in MCDS plays an active role in this arena.

Financial policies

The essence of the government's approach is to be compassionate in a way that will not rob the nation of its economic competitiveness. This is exemplified by the current design of financial protection for older Singaporeans — the Central Provident Fund. The CPF, a national social security fund, was established in 1955 as a form of retirement savings plan, which could be partially withdrawn at age 55. Employees under 55 years of age are required to save 20 per cent of their salary in a self-managed asset account, while their employers are also obliged to contribute 16 per cent into the employee's account. To make it more attractive for employers to employ older workers, the government has set a lower employers' contribution rate for employees who are 55 years of age and over (Table 5.2).

The CPF scheme has gradually evolved into "the world's most extensive social policy on assets" (Sherraden et al. 1995,

TABLE 5.2

Singapore: Percentage Rates of Central Provident Fund (CPF) Contributions for Employers and Employees (January 2001)

Age (in years)	Employer's Contribution (% of wage/salary)	Employee's Contribution (% of wage/salary)
Below 55	16.0	20.0
56–60	4.0	12.5
61–65	2.0	7.5
65 and above	2.0	5.0

Source: CPF Website: <www.cpf.gov.sg>

p. 112). Each working Singaporean has a CPF account, compartmentalized into the ordinary, special and Medisave accounts. Within certain limits, the individual can expend a portion of his or her savings on investments, housing, tertiary education for a child, and even home protection. The last is a "compulsory mortgage-reducing plan (which) protects members and their families from loss of their homes when members die or are permanently disabled" (Sherraden 1997, p. 42). Medisave is a compulsory hospitalization insurance scheme; Medishield is an optional low-cost catastrophic illness insurance; and the Dependents Protection scheme is an optional term-life insurance scheme which covers members for an insured sum until they reach the age of 60. All three schemes cover not only the individual but also his or her family. The CPF scheme has been criticized for its lack of universal coverage and the lack of adequacy of funds for retirement security, especially for the low-income groups (Shantakumar 1999; Asher 1996 and 1998; Lee 1999 and 2001*a*). The recent National Survey of Senior Citizens 1995 showed that only 33.5 per cent of those above the age of 60 had CPF savings and, of these, 61.6 per cent felt that their CPF savings were inadequate. The main reasons cited for inadequate security were high cost of living, low savings, and high medical costs. Children were the main source of financial support for the majority of the respondents in the survey (Ministry of Health et al., Singapore 1996). In line with its emphasis on family support, an aged dependent relief is provided under the income tax assessment. A co-residential child/child-in-law is eligible for S$5,000 tax relief annually, while the non-co-residential counterpart is eligible for S$3,500 annually, (US$1 = approximately S$1.80).

Apart from the CPF, there are two other schemes that act as a "safety net" for elderly Singaporeans. The first, a Public/Social Assistance scheme, is disbursed by the MCDS. The eligibility criteria are very stringent, and older persons with living children usually have a very slim chance of obtaining approval. The rates are not commensurate with Singapore's rising inflation; for example, an adult can obtain a maximum monthly allowance of only S$230 (about US$135). However, a person on Public Assistance is also entitled to free medical services, which is of great help. Secondly, the Medifund scheme is available for poor patients who are unable to pay their hospital bills. However, the onus for applying for this aid is on the patient, and sometimes they are not aware of its existence.

From the outset, the state opted for a non-welfare state approach and is reluctant to make cash payments directly to needy persons. This Singapore-style welfare strategy has been called "supply-side socialism" (*Straits Times*, 18 September 1994), in which any form of financial assistance is usually provided at source — for example, to the Housing Development Board for people in rent arrears, or to a nursing home to subsidize frail aged people. The rationale for this approach is to reduce the temptation of abuse by the recipient or his/her family members.

Health policies

In the arena of health care, Singapore has designed a system of subsidy for hospital beds under which Class C patients receive an 80 per cent subsidy, Class B2 patients receive a 65 per cent subsidy, and Class B1 patients receive a 20 per cent subsidy. The subsidy for nursing home beds has been revised following the recommendations of the report of the Inter-Ministerial Committee on Health Care for the Elderly in 1999. The philosophy adopted by the state is that each individual is responsible for maintaining his or her health and well-being, and should save for a rainy day. If this fails, the family should help out; the government will only come in as a last resort. A great deal of money is therefore being spent by the government on life-long public health education, as was seen in the recent announcement of the establishment of a statutory board, the Health Promotion Board (*Straits Times* 23 February 2001). This is a logical follow-up of the recommendation of the IMC on Health Care for the Elderly on the establishment of a national disability prevention programme.

Another dimension of primary health care, on which the government is focusing, is subsidized health screening for senior citizens. For a nominal fee of S$5, a person aged over 60 can access a basic health-screening test. This service has been promoted by the Ministry of Health using neighbourhood organizations, such as community centres/clubs as venues. The IMC Report on Ageing Population has also highlighted the importance of a comprehensive system of "step-down care" after a patient is discharged from hospital (Figure 5.2 summarizes the services).

FIGURE 5.2
Singapore: The Concept of Step-Down Care

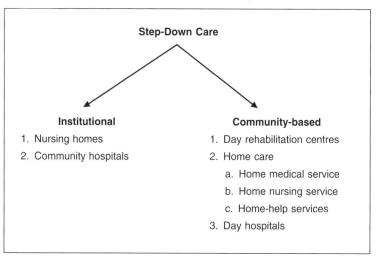

Source: Based on Inter-Ministerial Committee on the Ageing Population (1999).

While some of these services are presently available, inadequacy, unequal geographical distribution and affordability remain major issues. Linked to this topic is the need for more supportive programmes at the neighbourhood level to assist families in caring for their elderly members. Such programmes could include meal delivery, help-line telephone services, equipment loans, "elder minding" and even neighbourhood respite care. It is hoped that a viable network of such integrated services can prevent premature institutionalization. A continuum of care for sick older persons, from acute to community-based to home care, is the aim of the Singapore Government's policy for the older Singaporean, although this has yet to be achieved.

Housing policies

Through the Housing and Development Board (HDB), which is a statutory board, the Singaporean state has socially engineered children either to live together or to live within a short distance of their elderly parents and/or parents-in-law. "In 2000, about nine in 10 elderly persons above sixty five years and over lived with their spouse or children" (Government of Singapore 2000, p. 5). In their four-nation comparison of living arrangements of elderly persons aged 60 and over, Knodel and Debavalya (1997) found that the percentage of elderly people living with their children was highest in Singapore compared with the Philippines, Thailand and Vietnam. Elsewhere in the region, for example in Korea (Choi and Suh 1995) and Japan (Yamasaki 1999), the decline of co-residential living arrangements among older persons is an established trend.

The high rate of co-residence of older Singaporeans is probably explained by various housing schemes to encourage extended family living; the high cost of housing, given the scarcity of land area; and the cultural inclination towards filial care. It is not possible to describe all the housing schemes in this chapter, so selected examples will be cited. Among these, the Multi-Tier Housing Scheme gives priority allocation to extended-family applicants, and the Joint Selection Scheme is designed to allow families to select flats on priority so that married children and parents can stay in separate HDB flats but in close proximity. The CPF Housing Grant Scheme allows a married first-time applicant who buys a resale flat from the open market in order to stay near his or her parents or vice versa, to apply for a housing grant ranging between S$30,000– S$40,000, depending on the geographical proximity between the two generations. Apart from these examples, there are other housing schemes, such as the Joint MCDS-HDB Project, which is equipped with elderly-friendly facilities. This is targeted at low-income elderly people in rented one-room flats in which modifications such as non-slip tiles, lift landings on every floor and an alarm system have been installed at no cost to the resident. A Studio Apartment Scheme is aimed at elderly HDB flat-owners aged 50 and above who wish to downsize from larger to smaller elderly-friendly flats after retirement. In addition, the government provides funding to selected voluntary organizations to run activities for older persons within the ground floors of these selected blocks.

Likely future developments

The blueprint for future development of ageing policies in Singapore has been laid out in the two IMC Reports on Health Care for the Elderly (February 1999) and the Ageing Population (November 1999) which spans the recommendations of six work groups: Social Integration, Health Care, Financial Security, Employment and Employability, Housing and Land Use, and Cohesion and Conflict.

It is worth noting that a three-pronged approach was adopted towards achieving social integration: developing the "heartware" (positive attitudes and values towards older people), "software" (policies, programmes and services) and "hardware" (the built environment, including transport). On 12 January 2001, the minister for community development and sports outlined publicly for the first time the main features of the Five-Year Master Plan of Elder Care Services (*Straits Times*, 13 January 2001). Many of the points are logical concrete plans stemming from the recommendations of the two IMC reports. The three key strategies outlined in the master plan are:

1. The setting up of an appropriate infrastructure and a new service delivery system
2. The revamping of funding policy for voluntary elder care services
3. The provision of a continuum of programmes targeted at healthy older persons, frail elderly people and their caregivers.

Under the first strategy, multi-service centres, to meet the needs of different generations and managed by community development councils, would serve as one-stop centres. Multi-service centres would be complemented by Neighbourhood Link Centres, which would function as information dissemination and referral services while at the same time tapping the resources of healthy older persons and other age groups to engage in volunteer activities. Under the second strategy, from 1 April 2001, the funding for voluntary organizations was to involve subsidizing elderly-related services on a per capita basis rather than on a programme basis, wherever possible. A differential subsidy scale was to be introduced so that lower-income users would receive a higher subsidy. A competitive system of bidding for funds to operate a service was also expected to be launched.

Out of a total of S$93 million allocated towards the master plan, more than S$30 million was to be used for programmes for fit elderly people. A case management service was to be launched for frail elderly persons to facilitate accessibility to multiple services. Last, a formal commitment was made by the government to establish carer centres, in acknowledgement of the physical and emotional stress of caring for elder relatives and to provide family caregivers with information, training and recognition.

Apart from the outline developed by the minister, it is anticipated that Golden Manpower Centres, which offer training and employment opportunities for older Singaporeans, will be expanded. The relatively low labour force participation (LFP) rate of Singaporeans aged 55–60 years old is of concern to the government. The reasons lie in part in the low educational levels and lack of skills of older workers, as well as a lack of employment opportunities. The Golden Manpower Centres can help to mitigate the full impact of an ageing workforce on the economy. However, it is paradoxical that, while the retirement age has been gradually increased from 60 to 62 as of January 1999, the labour force participation rate of older workers has not increased much. In 1997, the LFP rate for the age group 55–64 was 43 per cent, markedly low as compared to their counterparts in Japan (67 per cent), Korea (64 per cent) and Hong Kong (52 per cent) (Inter-Ministerial Committee on Ageing Population, 1999).

To succeed, the government will have to work on the mindsets of both older workers and employers, in addition to providing incentives to employees to remain in the labour force. It is hoped that future cohorts of older persons, who are expected to be better educated than those of today, may be more inclined to continue working beyond 55 years of age. However, as seniority wages may work against their continued employment, a flexible, performance-based rather than seniority-based remuneration system is needed to deal with this challenge.

Last, Eldershield, an insurance scheme related to disability in old age, was introduced on 30 September 2002. The premiums are deducted from the Medisave portion of a CPF policy holder's account and, in the event of at least one ADL disability, he/she is eligible to apply for a subsidy of S$300 per month for a maximum period of 5 years. The premiums are higher for women than men as a result of their longer life expectancy. The coverage is for life and premiums have to be paid between the ages of 45 to 65, unless a Singaporean voluntarily opts out (for more details, see website <www.cpf.gov.sg>).

Long-term care (LTC)

It may be pondered whether there will really be a pressing need for long-term care facilities, given that a relatively high number of elderly people in Singapore live with their family members. Indeed, according to the National Survey of Senior Citizens 1995, 86.2 per cent lived with their children, an increase of about 5 per cent from 1983. The survey also reported that 3.1 per cent of senior citizens lived alone, while another 5.2 per cent lived with their spouse only (Ministry of Health et al., Singapore 1996). The survey was national, covering a sample of 4,750 older persons and achieving a 50 per cent response rate. Subsequently, the Singapore Census of Population 2000 recorded an increase in "elderly only" households from 1.8 per cent in 1990 to 2.8 per cent in 1999. Parallel to this trend, there was also a decrease of extended or multi-generational households from 6.7 per cent to 5.6 per cent. The census also documented an increase in one-person households from 5.2 per cent in 1990 to 8.2 per cent in 1999 (Table 5.3).

TABLE 5.3
Singapore: Changes in Household Structure, 1980–2000

Household Structure	1980	1990	2000
% of one-person households	5.7	5.2	8.2
% of one family nuclear households	81.0	84.6	82.1
% of multi-family nuclei household	10.8	6.7	5.6

Source: Department of Statistics Singapore (2001).

The increase of 3 per cent in one-person households is a matter of concern due to the potential of social isolation, vulnerability to depression and suicide, as well as the lower possibility of immediate treatment at times of crisis. While a healthy older person may not have much difficulty in managing to live independently, frail or handicapped older persons are far more likely to need formal and informal assistance.

Other demographics affecting the need for long-term care are:

The ageing of the aged population. In Singapore, this follows the trend in many other countries (Kinsella 2000) in which the rate of increase of the "oldest-old" population (people aged over 75) is greater than that of the "young-old" population (60–65 year olds). A consequence of this demographic transformation appears to be a substantial increase in the utilization of health care services. In 1995, for example, people aged 65 and over accounted for only

7 per cent of the population but totalled 17 per cent of all hospital admissions and 19 per cent of out-patient polyclinic visits (Phua and Yap 1998). These statistics have alerted health care policy-makers in planning for future demands.

Older women.   The feminization of ageing is a common feature that reflects the gender bias in the numbers of older women surviving as compared to older men in very old populations, given women's advantage in terms of life expectancy. Although this can be seen as a neutral demographic feature, health statistics show that women tend to suffer more from chronic illnesses while men tend to be inflicted by acute or fatal illnesses such as cardio-vascular disease (Muller 1992). The net result is that in many countries women often require physical assistance due to illnesses such as arthritis, rheumatism and asthma. Longer life expectancy, chronic illness, and quite often inadequate financial resources accentuate the needs of older women for LTC (Lee 2001*a*). In Singapore, women outnumber men in nursing homes. The lack of research data on ageing women per se is a gap that needs to be addressed in Singapore, as in many other developed countries.

In Singapore, Shantakumar's monograph 1994 based on 1990 census data highlighted that "frail widowed elderly women would be significant among the future aged, with attendant problems of financial security, medical and health supports" (p. 50). Parallel to this it should also be remembered that a considerable proportion of middle-aged and elderly women provide care to older relatives, such as spouses, parents and parents-in-law. Indeed, it has been suggested that women can expect to spend as much time caring for an ageing parent as raising children (Clair et al 2000), so the lifetime cumulative negative costs of this in terms of finance, physical and mental health, and lost opportunities are experienced by most women at old age. Women almost everywhere comprise the majority of informal family caregivers to older persons, including in Singapore (Mehta 2000). Recent research in the Singapore context has documented the stress faced by female spouses in the caregiving role (Mehta and Joshi 2000). However, more optimistically, the likelihood of better education and longer careers may benefit future cohorts of women in developing countries when they reach old age.

Lonely older persons.   Lonely people, be they male or female, often require social networks to maintain their integration with the rest of the society. Indeed, the well-being of older people is closely linked with the availability of social support, a key point that has been emphasized by many social researchers (Antonucci 1990; Argyle 1992). A clear trend surfacing in the demographic statistics of Singapore is the increase in single males and females. For the age group 40–44, the number of single male Singaporeans increased by about 5 per cent between 1990 and 2000 (from 10.4 to 15.5 per cent) while the commensurate increase for females was 3 per cent (from 11.4 to 14.1 per cent) (Department of Statistics, Singapore 2001). Although the possibility of marriage after the age of 45 cannot be excluded, the chances are usually slimmer. At the risk of sounding pessimistic, it is highly possible that loneliness could be a common experience of single men and women in old age, unless they prepare for this by servicing friendships and maintaining ties with siblings, cousins and other relatives.

Financing of long-term care

The financing of LTC is a complex area because it is interwoven with the total health care delivery system. Unarguably, Singapore has made considerable progress in the provision of health care and, in comparison to many other developing countries, it has a comprehensive health care system accessible to all Singaporeans (Smith 1994). In the early 1990s, a review of health care policies identified the need for cost containment of health care expenditure and the government's role in provision of secondary and tertiary care. One of the key recommendations in the main report of the review was:

> The (Singapore) Government should take the lead to implement a comprehensive programme for the care of the elderly sick. This includes the provision of more hospital beds for geriatric care, nursing homes, day care

and respite facilities, and home support services. The private sector, voluntary organizations and general practitioners should be encouraged to participate in this programme. (Ministry of Health, Singapore 1992, p. ix).

Although the health care system targets all Singaporeans regardless of age, this report emphasized the needs of elderly people.

Continuing care is seen as addressing issues from a global perspective relating to all aspects of health and social service systems continuing care is not, therefore a type of service as such, but a system of service delivery. (Hennessy 1996, p. 4).

The term "continuing care" is increasingly popular in some countries, indicating the appreciation that physical health and social health are intricately connected — which is especially true with regard to services for older persons. Indeed, Evashwick (1996) stresses that a continuum of care should be client-oriented and emphasize "wellness" rather than illness. An effective comprehensive array of elderly care services in any country would have to acknowledge the blending of heath and social services and, in Singapore as in many other countries, as noted in Chapter 1, the term "seamless" in health care delivery systems is gaining popularity with policy-makers and service providers. As a complement to acute care, the concept of step-down-care has been developed.

With the entry of the baby boomers' cohort, the shape of the population pyramid is slowly changing into a pillar, and policy-makers have recognized the pressing need for an integrated system of long-term care. The major question is, as ever, who will pay for these services? In Singapore, government policy has been that the financial responsibility for older people lies with the individual, the family, the community and, lastly, the state (Phillips and Bartlett 1995; Smith 1994; Teo 1994). The state has also set up Medifund, a fund which provides financial assistance to patients who cannot afford their hospitalization bills, and an Elder Care Fund to finance the operations of nursing homes run by voluntary welfare organizations (*Straits Times*, 24 August 2000). It can be seen, therefore, that the funding of health and social care services to date has been via a combination of sources: individuals (and indirectly, employers), the family, voluntary welfare institutions and the state. A safety net exists for those who do not have any family, in the form of Public Assistance from the government, the Medifund scheme and various charitable organizations.

Current provision and developments in long-term care

Here, "long-term care", which has many different interpretations, is used, as defined in Chapter 1, to include the full range of health, personal care and social services provided at home and in the community for a continuing period to adults who lack or have lost the capacity to care fully for themselves and to remain independent (Phillips 2000). In Singapore, as in most other countries in the region, there was relatively little debate or discussion on the topic of LTC until recently, as families were assumed to be the long-term care providers. Those without families, or the destitute, were dependent on the state for shelter and their material needs. Non-governmental organizations, such as religious bodies and ethnic associations, were commonly found to care for those who either did not succeed in obtaining government assistance or who preferred to cope without the state's help due to pride, fear of stigmatization and other reasons. Unlike many non-Asian countries, where government assistance is viewed as an entitlement, in Singapore the general sentiment is that one only applies for the state's help when one has no other options available. To many, it signals "failure" in life. Yet, as discussed in Chapter 1, in much of Asia, the family is no longer able to continue to take care of elderly members, because of the limited human and financial resources available to a smaller family, even if there is no convincing evidence that there is an erosion of family values (Liu and Kendig 2000; Ng et al. 2002).

The ageing of aged populations in many countries, as well as shrinking of the pool of traditional caregivers such as daughters and daughters-in-law, has fuelled the growing concern over LTC.

In Singapore, an additional factor is the high cost of medical care, especially with regard to hospitalization.

Current provisions for long-term care as of January 2001 in Singapore comprise:

Residential LTC: hospitals for the chronically ill: for long-stay patients (2); community hospitals for rehabilitation after an acute illness (4); nursing homes (47); hospices (3); homes for dementia patients (2); cluster living or studio apartments (6 blocks); and the joint HDB-MCDS housing project (25 blocks).

Non-Residential LTC: day rehabilitation centres (23); social day care centres (11); day-care centres for dementia patients (3); and home care, such as home medical care, home nursing care and home help.

Community-based support services.   These include meal delivery services; laundry services; home modification services — for example, installation of grab bars, non-slip tiles and levelled floors; a telephone hotline service, for crisis and counselling; a befriender service, where volunteers are matched with lonely elderly people for home visits; mutual help groups — neighbourhood-based small groups of about 10–30 older persons to foster mutual care and concern; escort services, for volunteers to accompany elderly to clinics or hospital; bereavement and funeral services, where volunteers offer help to bereaved families with funeral arrangements, or arrange funerals for the destitute elderly; and an alarm response service, where staff at a voluntary organization in the vicinity respond to an elderly resident's call for help when the alarm is used.

The rest of this section discusses these provisions in greater detail, including their limitations and future demands.

Residential long-term care

The IMC Report on Health Care for the Elderly pointed out that the demand for nursing homes far outstrips the supply (Inter-Ministerial Committee on Health Care for the Elderly 1999). It has been an unspoken policy in Singapore that nursing homes should be controlled in order not to encourage family members to turn to them as a first resort. The rationale has been that family care would be affected negatively if there was easy availability of institutional nursing home care. This policy has been modified after the Inter-Ministerial Committee on Ageing Population (1999) completed its analysis of data collection and feedback.

Table 5.4 summarizes the projected gap between the demand and supply of residential and community-based long-term care services from 1997 to 2030. From these data, it is apparent that there is and will be a shortage of facilities in almost every category. In particular, hospital beds for chronically ill persons, community hospital beds, home nursing, home medical and home-help services urgently need to be increased to avert a dramatic outcry from the public for long-term care services.

The government provides subventions (grants in aid) to voluntary welfare organizations that operate nursing homes and sheltered homes (which do not provide nursing/medical care). The Ministry of Health provides 90 per cent of the capital funding costs of nursing homes, and 50 per cent of operating expenditures, calculated on a per patient basis, with the actual amount fixed by the category of patient.[1]

To encourage the establishment of more private nursing homes, the government has announced that it will be releasing 17 sites for tender for private companies wishing to set up nursing homes (*Straits Times*, 21 May 2001). Due to the very high costs of land, a commodity in short supply in Singapore, the private companies will however need to target middle-income and upper-income groups of older Singaporeans.

The Elder Care Fund, set up in 2000, has been approved for funding the entire range of elderly and continuing care facilities, including nursing homes, community hospitals, hospices, day rehabilitation, home medical and home nursing services. The state has injected an initial sum of S$200 million which will be increased to S$2.5 billion by 2010. Budget surpluses will be used to build up the capital in this endowment fund specially created to help subsidize lower-and lower- middle-class Singaporeans.

In addition to funding, the fragmented nature of the health and long-term care system has been noted in Singapore, and it

TABLE 5.4
Singapore: Projected Needs for Health Services for Older Persons, 2000–30

Types of Service	Planning Ratio Caps	1997	2000	2010	2020	2030
			Year			
Acute-care geriatric beds	1 bed per 1,000 elderly	217 (188)	235 [226]	310	530	800
Geriatric specialist	1 specialist per 10,000 elderly	22 (15)	25 [21]	30	55	80
Community hospital beds	3.5 beds per 1,000 elderly	761 (426)	820 [426]a	1,090	1,855	2,800
Sick hospital beds for the chronically ill	1.5 beds per 1,000 elderly	326 (218)	352 [218]a	480	800	1,200
Nursing home beds (including beds for dementia patients)	28 beds per 1,000 elderly	6,087 (4,703)	6,566 [5,635]a	8,800	14,900	22,400
Day rehabilitation and day care places (including places for dementia patients)	3.5 places for 1,000 elderly	761 (701)	821 [820]	1,100	1,900	2,800
Home medical care service (projection unit: home medical care units per month)	5 elderly needing 1 visit per month per 1,000 elderly	1,087 (750)	1,173 [825]	1,600	2,700	4,000
Home nursing service (projection unit: home nursing units per month)	15 elderly needing 2 visits per month per 1,000 elderly	6,522 (5,000)	7,035 [5,500]	9,400	15,900	24,000
Home-help service (projection unit: number of home help visits per day)	4 elderly needing daily visits per 1,000 elderly	870 (255)	938 [300]	1,250	2,120	3,200

Note: ( ) = Availability in 1997.
[ ] = Estimated availability in 2000.
a Estimated availability will improve by 2003: chronic sick hospital beds for the chronically ill (400); nursing home beds (7,300).
Source: Inter-Ministerial Committee on Health Care for the Elderly (1999).

creates hurdles for potential clients and their families in accessing services. To address this, the Ministry of Health in the early 2000s, announced a framework for integrated healthcare services for the elderly, to be put in place over the next ten years. The needs of older persons change over time; for example, someone who is in one facility such as a day-care centre may later need more intensive health care services after a fall or accident. According to the framework, Singapore's acute and step-down community-based services will be divided into three geographical zones (West, Central and East) and there will be close networking within each zone for patients' benefit.

Another attempt to address the problem of fragmentation of services is via the introduction of the case management service. The National Council of Social Service, a statutory body, launched a two-year pilot project in May 1998 in collaboration with two non-profit organizations, the Singapore Action Group of Elders (SAGE) and the Tsao Foundation. SAGE views case management as a new service which involves the assessment of an elderly person's health, psychological and social needs and the maximization of services to attain the optimal and most cost-effective care of the elderly and their caregivers to prevent unnecessary institutionalization. This strategy of service delivery is being expanded in order to mitigate the problems of the uneven distribution of services and fragmentation in service delivery. The aim is to develop viable models of case management to suit the Singapore context.

Non-residential long-term care and support services
Although there is a wide array of community-based services available, as noted above, with the exception of the home nursing service, all are inadequate given the demand. Moreover, services are unevenly distributed across the island, so family members may have to travel long distances to reach a particular service; older persons will similarly need to travel for long periods, causing fatigue. If the government policy of "ageing in place" is to be successful, more day-care centres will have to be established in all housing estates with relevant support services, so that the needs of families with ageing members are met in a comprehensive way. Anecdotal evidence relates that older

persons are sometimes left to sit in public spaces for long hours while their children and grandchildren are away at work or school, which highlights the need for local day-care and social drop-in centres. Greater use could be made of family service centres (of which there were 31 in April 2001) to accommodate the needs of senior citizens. Within the programmes, day-care centre staff could be better trained not only to be sensitive to the needs of older people but also to be innovative, for example organizing mentally stimulating activities such as autobiography and reminiscence group sessions. However staff at present do not have to undergo training and, indeed, training courses are few and far between. The National Council of Social Service, the umbrella body coordinating all voluntary welfare organizations, has a training department which organizes talks and workshops on an ad hoc basis for staff. However, many staff lack the motivation to attend, as they do not see the direct benefits of attendance except for gaining a certificate of attendance. A training centre set up by the Tsao Foundation is another resource for organizing training for staff of day-care centres and homes for elderly persons.[2]

Challenges ahead

Issues of coordination

Most of the community-based long-term social care facilities fall under the auspices of the Ministry of Community Development and Sports (MCDS), while nursing home facilities, hospices, community and hospitals for the chronically ill are under the Ministry of Health (MOH).[3] Although the Inter-Ministerial Committee on Ageing Population, now a standing committee housed under the MCDS, has addressed some of the problems of coordination, the situation is not ideal. The crux of this problem is that services for the aged are multi-disciplinary and older people's issues are multi-dimensional. Australia, for one, has addressed this by creating a Ministry for the Aged, while some other countries have combined the Ministry of Health and Welfare, as in Japan. In the field of long-term care for older people, the Singapore Government should address the pressing need for close coordination between the two ministries, perhaps by appointing a senior official to be assigned this special portfolio.

Personnel issues

The availability of appropriate personnel is a major issue facing voluntary welfare organizations, as they generally operate on lean budgets and volunteers may not easily be recruited, a situation common in many countries (Kleunen and Wilner 2001). In Singapore, under 10 per cent of citizens volunteer their services and the majority are in religious and community service activities (Ho and Chua 1990). When this is compared to the United States, for example, where an estimated 40 per cent of the population is involved in voluntary activities, it becames clear that there is room for promoting a culture of volunteerism in Singapore. Retirees and housewives form a potential resource to supplement and complement the roles of staff in LTC facilities. In Australia, for example, middle-aged and older Australians have been found to comprise the majority of volunteers (Encel and Nelson 1996). One possible explanation for the low levels of voluntary participation by older Singaporeans is the active role and functions played by older Singaporeans in their families as grandparents, which leaves them little time for community involvement. A second reason may be that many have low levels of education; in 1995, 89.2 per cent of people aged 65–74 years had only primary level education or below (Inter-Ministerial Committee on Ageing Population 1999). The low levels of education often imply a lack of English language fluency and often a lack of confidence in being able to help others. The Retired and Senior Volunteers Programme (RSVP) has a branch in Singapore, and it is hoped that it will succeed in recruiting a larger pool of senior volunteers to contribute to the voluntary services industry.

Issues of professional assessment

Despite the efforts of various community groups and individuals, and the planning of services for the elderly with the vision of achieving an age-integrated society, a major shortcoming remains the lack of attention to standardized procedures for geriatric assessment. The standardization of geriatric assessment protocol across all hospitals, nursing homes, day-care centres and community sheltered homes should be viewed as part of the process of the professionalization of care for older persons in Singapore. Without this, a variety of instruments and protocol will result in inconsistent health assessments and delayed admission, causing services to be inefficient. Singapore could benefit by studying, for example, the Minimum Data Set-Home Care Version 2 (MDS-HC) introduced by Hong Kong in 2000 as a "gate-keeping mechanism" for older persons applying to residential and community-based services (Yuen 2001). Another model that could be examined for application in the Singapore context is the support needs assessment protocol (SNAP) used in New Zealand (Howe 1996). The advantages of having such a standardized protocol include avoiding the duplication of time and effort, and transfers between facilities are made more efficient. At present, when an elderly patient is discharged from an acute hospital and a medical social worker applies to a nursing home, the home applies its own assessment procedure, which sometimes can take a couple of weeks. This leads to negative outcomes such as family anxiety and arguments over caring arrangements, professional frustration among medical social workers and staff of residential and community-based facilities, and often depression and sadness on the part of the older person who feels responsible for the family's turmoil.

Recent developments such as the inter-ministerial committee reports and the unveiling of the Five-Year Master Plan of Elder Care Services (under the Elderly Development Division, MCDS) have to some extent addressed the question of what physical facilities are likely to be required over the next few decades. Recommendations have been made to improve the current financing options for LTC services, but not enough emphasis has been placed on issues relating to practice. Some of these practice issues include the need for relevant training and incentives for staff of LTC facilities, standardization of procedures and protocol for assessment of older clients, coordination between agencies providing LTC to reduce administration and improve efficiency, and the monitoring of the quality of LTC facilities.

The Ministry of Health is responsible for monitoring the quality of care in nursing homes, which include homes for dementia patients. Imaginative programmes could go a long way to improving the lives of dementia patients and their caregivers (Hartz and Splain 1997; Burgio et al. 2000). Issues related to the effective management of residential homes for older adults are highlighted by Langlais (1997), especially in relation to increasing staff commitment and enthusiasm.

Quality of care is intrinsically also related to sensitivity to the cultural and religious needs of residents. These may include dietary preferences, language and communication, preferences for dressing, and music and prayer requirements. Many cultural sensitivities also involve the meaning of death, end-of-life issues and preferences of older residents with regard to funerals and religious rituals. These are all extremely relevant in LTC facilities such as hospices, hospitals for the chronically ill and geriatric counselling services, especially in a multicultural society such as Singapore (Mui et al. 1998; Kagawa-Singer 1994). At the very old and often terminal stage of their lives, older adults may be subjected to a succession of admissions and discharges followed by re-admissions to acute/chronic care facilities. Culturally sensitive environments would go a long way to reduce the trauma of these successive entries and exits. Managers of LTC facilities should be inculcated with the importance of this ingredient of quality care in their training programmes.

Areas for policy development

The Singapore Government has clearly spelt out the aims of the Five-Year Master Plan of Elder Care Services: to promote the social integration of older Singaporeans and to ensure a more integrated delivery of elder care services at the community level. This reflects the philosophy of the state that older persons should be encouraged to be active and continue to be part of society's mainstream. The rest of the measures, such as those to help people remain within their families and communities by attending retraining programmes and preventive life-long health education, are consistent with this approach. The second main thrust of the policies is to encourage self-reliance and family interdependence, in keeping with the self-dignity and family-oriented nature of Asian cultures.

The overall policy design for older Singaporeans is sound in concept although, in reality, the demographic trends reveal a rise in the numbers of single adults, which signals a possible lack of family support in old age. "During 1990–1995, the proportion of singles increased for each of the age group 20–44 except those aged 30–34" (Department of Statistics, Singapore 1995, p. 6). The number of divorces has also risen across the board for all ethnic groups, and with social trends signalling a rise in single and divorced adults, there is a need for revision of policies to consider their needs and, for example, to provide incentives for siblings to care for one another.

Advocacy by older persons

The literacy rate for resident Singaporeans above the age of 15 has risen from 89 per cent in 1990 to 93 per cent in 2000 (Singapore Cesus of Population 2000), and rising educational levels are seen with each successive cohort of elderly Singaporeans (Table 5.5). A greater advocacy role should therefore be provided to middle-aged and older Singaporeans. Establishing channels for older persons to provide input into policy initiatives is healthy and can help to ensure that the implementation of policies is effective and matched with the needs of successive cohorts. In this way,

TABLE 5.5

**Singapore: Education Profile of Persons Aged 65–74,
1995 and Estimates to 2030**

Educational	1995		2010		2030	
Qualifications	No.	%	No.	%	No.	%
Primary & below	116,403	89.2	139,600	71.2	191,200	37.8
Secondary	8,989	6.9	32,100	16.4	161,100	31.8
Upper secondary[a]	3,314	2.5	16,700	8.5	87,600	17.3
University	1,776	1.4	7,600	3.9	66,500	13.1
Total	**130,482**	**100.0**	**196,000**	**100.0**	**506,400**	**100.0**

[a] Includes polytechnic graduates.
Source: Inter-Ministerial Committee on the Ageing Population (1999).

there will probably be less wastage of resources and a bridge built between service providers and recipients.

Singapore is also becoming an increasingly affluent society and, inevitably, there will be associated social costs. "The median household income from work grew from S$2,300 in 1990 to S$3,600 in 2000. In real terms, the median household income grew by 2.8 per cent" (Singapore Census of Population, Data Release 9). Since there is no official poverty line and no comprehensive national database on the poor, identifying this group in Singapore and compiling the statistics is difficult. Nevertheless, "it has been predicted that a potential underclass from a developed Singapore may come from three risk groups" (Low and Ngiam 1999, p. 241). Two of these are older workers and non-working women, possibly older widows. According to the 1995 National Survey of Senior Citizens, the median monthly income of senior citizens was S$518, which is unarguably low. Given the social demographic scenario, coupled with the lack of universal coverage of the CPF scheme and the fact that many older workers have been laid off in the recession (*Straits Times* 7 August 2000), some revision of policy initiatives is called for. Although safety nets do exist, they will not be able to cater for rising numbers of older persons who fall at the borderline, or face a temporary crisis such as being retrenched, or who do not have children to maintain them. The standardized approach to policies on ageing needs to be revamped, paving the way for greater refinement and customized policy provisions as times change and new scenarios emerge.

Within ageing and the aged policies arena in Singapore, there is a need for more research in certain specific areas. For example, one area is the implementation of retraining packages for older workers and the causes of their low uptake. If financial subsidies are not effective, other factors have to be examined, such as the delivery of the training packages or the poor response from potential employers of older workers, which could explain the lack of popularity of the retraining schemes. There is quite a lot of innovative research in some other areas; for example, there is ongoing research on menopause and its impact on the lives of older women. There is also a national survey on male ageing patterns within a sample of 1,000 males aged between

45–70 years. The aim of the latter study is to study andropause and its effects on Asian males.

Support and programmes for family caregivers

In view of increasing medical costs and hospitalization expenses, policy-makers should revise the aged dependency relief for co-residential children and children-in-law. The current annual income tax relief for this group is S$5,000, which works out to a mere S$375 per month. Moreover, it has been noted by the IMC on Ageing Population (1999) that a large majority of families may not benefit from this relief because their income bracket is too low, so a means-tested subsidy in lieu of tax relief would probably benefit these family caregivers. If it is agreed that the economic burden of care for older persons falls unevenly on lower-income families, then such a subsidy should be supported and implemented without delay. It might encourage children to continue caregiving and it could also reduce the incidence of abuse due to the financial stress of caring for elderly parents. In general, it is clear that a great deal more needs to be done both in policy formulation and implementation for the translation of the recommendations of the IMC reports into reality.

Creation of a barrier-free society

The physical environment and infrastructure often need modification to achieve barrier-free status. "Older people often apologise because they are unable to use the built environment anymore — but it is the built environment (and more especially its creators) who should be apologising to these older people for its inadequacy or hostility" (Harrison 2001). The city–state of Singapore has room for improvement in creating a more elderly-friendly physical environment. A good starting point would be the reduction in the number of steps at entrances to facilities such as shopping malls and subway stations, and making the pavements gradual so that an electric wheelchair user can be independent.

Transport policies and policies in relation to education in the Third Age have also been under-emphasized. With the swiftly ageing demographic profile, and one which forecasts a more educated and relatively affluent population, mobility and opportunities for education in the post-retirement years will be important issues. Singaporean policy-makers have to study the rationale behind limiting things such as the bus concession times for senior citizens to off-peak hours (10 a.m.–4 p.m. and after 7 p.m.) and whether this constrains their contribution to society. Tertiary institutions could consider setting up summer courses for interested seniors, preceded by a needs assessment survey indicating the types of courses that would be popular. In this field, there is ample room for private sector involvement. Policy-makers need to be well prepared for a new generation of older persons in the next two decades, who will know and demand the well-deserved fruits of their labour, unlike many in the present generation who are humble and regard the state as the paternalistic authority.

Notes

1. There are four categories of patients using the Resident Assessment Form (RAF) which assesses the physical and mental needs of potential residents and their dependence on nursing care and assistance for the activities of daily living (ADLs). Category 1 is the least functionally dependent and Category 4 the most dependent.
2. Further information is available on the websites of the Tsao Foundation:<www.tsaofoundation.org> and the National Council of Social Service: <www.ncss.org.sg>.
3. The Homes for the Aged Bill was passed in 1988. It stipulates that these homes must be licensed and comply with the guidelines on minimum standards of care for their residents. Sub-standard homes would be required to close down if they fail to meet the standards after a reasonable period of time after warning.

   The Ministry of Health regulates day-care centres and nursing homes under the Private Hospitals and Medical Clinics Act. The guidelines include space requirements, standard facilities, furnishings and equipment, and staffing, although neither address the minimum requirements of training in elder care.

6

National Policies on Ageing and Long-term Care Provision for Older Persons in Thailand

Sutthichai Jitapunkul,
Napaporn Chayovan and
Jiraporn Kespichayawattana

Introduction

Thailand is currently experiencing among the most rapid rates of population ageing in the developing world and, given that demographic ageing in Thailand is a recent occurrence, there has been very little time to cope with its consequences. Hence, it is imperative that Thailand has a well-prepared national policy and programme on ageing as well as for long-term care services for the elderly. This chapter begins with an overview of the ageing situation in Thailand, followed by a description of the first National Long-term Plan for the elderly, the major programmes developed and the national policies on ageing in the Second National Long-term Plan for Older Persons. The chapter then aims to clarify the current situation with respect to long-term care in Thailand, the need for long-term care and the development of long-term care policy and provision.

National policy on ageing

The present situation of population ageing in Thailand

Whilst the number of older persons in Asia and the Pacific region, including Thailand, is expected to rise dramatically over the next decade, a more important issue for Thailand is the speed of its population ageing.

FIGURE 6.1

Thailand: Number and Percentage of Population Aged 60 Years and Over, 1960–2020

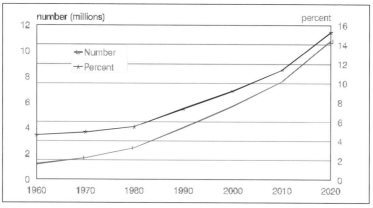

Source: Jitapunkul and Bunnag (1997).

Figure 6.1 shows that in 1990 the share of the elderly population aged 60 years and over was 7 per cent (5.6 million) and reached 9 per cent (6.2 million) in 2000. By 2020, the proportion of the elderly population is predicted to rise to 15 per cent, at which time the elderly cohorts will number more than 7 million (Jitapunkul et al. 2001). The speed of population ageing in Thailand is much faster than in many developed countries. For example, while it took England and Wales 107 years for the proportion of older persons (age 60 and over) to double from 7 per cent to 14 per cent, this will take Thailand only 30 years (Jitapunkul and Bunnag 1997). The rapid speed of population ageing in Thailand will have subsequent consequences for its socio-economic development, demanding timely and well-planned policies and programmes.

Given the rapid rate of population ageing, Thailand will have relatively a short period of time to deal with the consequences of these demographic changes.

Whilst they are imperfect measures, dependency ratios can give an indication of the potential burden of support on the working-age population. These ratios include the child dependency ratio (numbers of young people aged, say, 0–15 years relative to working–aged individuals aged 15–59) or the old-age dependency ratio (persons aged, say, 60 and above relative to working-aged individuals). The old-age ratio is clearly now rising. In 1960, for example, the total dependency ratio was 92 per 100 working population, and all of the dependent population were children. As birth rates declined, the child dependency ratio declined with an initial reduction of the total dependency ratio. Similarly, during the process of population ageing, the old age dependency ratio increased. The combination of the trends contributed to an initial reduction of the total dependency ratio, which will reach its nadir by 2010. Thereafter, the ratio will dramatically increase. According to a United Nations population projection, after 2026, the old-age dependency ratio in Thailand will be higher than the child dependency ratio (Figure 6.2).

FIGURE 6.2
**Thailand: Total, Child and Aged Dependency Ratios,
1950–2050 (per hundred)**

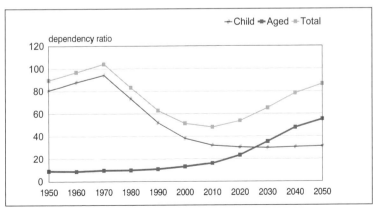

Source: Calculated from data in United Nations (1999*b*).

As in many other countries in the region, the role and structure of the family as well as in patterns of labour and migration in Thailand have undergone changes. Urbanization, the migration of young people to cities for employment, smaller family size, changing lifestyles, economic constraints and more women entering the workforce, mean that fewer people are available to care for older people when they are in need of assistance. Although family ties and support to aged parents are still strong and widely prevalent, their sustainability in the future is unclear, although they are currently holding up quite well (Knodel et al. 2000).

Inequities and the feminization of ageing exist in Thai society (Jitapunkul 1998a; Jitapunkul et al. 1999). Poor older people, particularly those living in rural areas, have suffered from the inequities and feminization of ageing by being further excluded from accessibility to health services, credit schemes, income-generating activities and decision-making (Table 6.1).

Although elderly women live longer than elderly men, it appears they spend more years with disabilities (Tables 6.2, 6.3 and 6.4). The ratios between health expectancy and life expectancy shown in Table 6.5 demonstrate that Thai men have a proportionally longer healthy life than do Thai women. While the importance of the gap between sexes in disability-free life expectancy (DFLE) seems to diminish with age, the proportional time of disability for both men and women increases with age.

Unfortunately, there is evidence from recent research suggesting that Thailand is in a stage of "morbidity expansion", in which age-specific rates of chronic diseases and disabilities are increasing (Jitapunkul et al. 1999; Jitapunkul 2000a). In addition, HIV/AIDS and drug addiction are also serious problems in Thailand and definitely have an impact on families, communities, and national health and social services and resource allocation, and hence on the older population.

With respect to the psychology of ageing, it may be said that Thai society is still stuck in an out-dated paradigm that considers old age as being associated with sickness, dependence and lack of productivity. However, by contrast, most people in Thailand do seem to adapt to change with age and remain independent

TABLE 6.1
Thailand: Characteristics of Elderly Women and Men Indicating a Vulnerable Situation for Elderly Women (percentages)

		Male			Female		
		Total	Urban	Rural	Total	Urban	Rural
Marital status	Single	1.1	1.3	1.1	3	5.2	2.4
	Married	83.3	85.6	82.7	48.9	42.8	50.4
	Widowed-divorced-separated	15.5	12.8	16.2	48	52	47.1
	Unknown	0.1	0.3	—	0.1	—	0.1
Education	None	19.4	14.4	20.6	40.9	33	42.7
	Less than grade 4	9.6	6.5	10.2	10.6	6.6	11.6
	Grade 4	59.5	47.3	62.3	44.3	45.2	44.1
	Higher than grade 4	10.7	30.9	6.1	3.8	14.5	1.3
	Others	0.8	0.9	0.8	0.4	0.7	0.3
Working status	Yes	41.8	29.4	44.5	23.8	16.6	25.6
Adequacy of income	Inadequate	37	21.3	40.5	34.1	18.6	37.8
Index of working opportunity (IWO)[a]	Ratio between "% working status as "yes" and "% inadequacy of income"	112.9	138	109.9	69.8	89.2	67.7

[a] A population with a high IWO means that the population has a high opportunity to work. This index is useful for comparing the opportunity to work or inequality of finding work among various populations.
Source: Jitapunkul (1998a).

TABLE 6.2
Thailand: Long-term Disability, Total Disability and Dependency in Self-Care Activities (percentages)

	Male				Female			
	All	60–69	70–79	80+	All	60–69	70–79	80+
Long-term disability[a]	17.4	14.6	19.4	27.6	20.2	14.9	23.4	36.0
Total disability[b]	22.0	19.5	22.9	33.3	27.2	22.7	30.6	39.7
Self-care Dependence[c]	5.7	4.0	5.4	16.1	7.9	4.4	8.9	20.9

[a] Long-term disability is defined as having limitations in any activities for six months or longer.
[b] Total disability is defined as having long-term disability or having no long-term disability but short-term disability (recent limitation of activities due to current illnesses).
[c] Self-care dependence is defined as being in need of help or supervision in any self-care activity of daily living, including feeding, grooming, transferring, toileting, dressing and bathing.
Source: Jitapunkul et al. (1999).

TABLE 6.3
Thailand: Severity of Long-term Disability by Age and Sex (percentages)

	Male				Female			
	All	60–69	70–79	80+	All	60–69	70–79	80+
Long-term disability[a]	17.4	14.6	19.4	27.6	20.2	14.9	23.4	36.0
Overall	17.4	14.6	19.4	27.6	20.2	14.9	23.4	36.0
Not home-bound	13.7	12.3	15.4	16.1	14.6	12.5	17.4	17.8
Home-bound	2.5	1.7	2.7	6.9	3.5	1.3	4.0	12.5
Chair/bed-bound	0.6	0.4	0.5	2.3	0.8	0.6	0.9	1.3
Totally dependent	0.6	0.2	0.7	2.3	1.2	0.5	1.1	4.4

Source: Jitapunkul et al. (1999).

well into very old age. A substantial proportion of older persons continue to work in paid and unpaid labour and, indeed, they are important resources for family support. Some older people are contributing to society by participating in voluntary activities.

As elsewhere in the region, since the Asian economic crisis of 1997, the economy of Thailand has been in a recovery period and

TABLE 6.4

Thailand: Life Expectancy and Disability-free Life Expectancy by age and sex (percentages)

	Male				Female			
	LE[a]	LDFLE[b]	TDFLE[c]	ALE[d]	LE	LDFLE	TDFLE	ALE
60–64	20.3	16.4	15.4	18.6	23.9	18.2	16.7	21.3
65–69	17.1	13.5	12.8	15.5	20.2	14.8	13.5	17.6
70–74	14.2	10.9	10.3	12.6	16.7	11.8	10.9	14.3
75–79	11.9	9.0	8.4	10.4	14.6	9.8	9.1	12.0
80+	10.9	7.9	7.3	9.0	13.6	8.7	8.2	10.8

[a] Life expectancy.
[b] Long-term disability-free life expectancy.
[c] Total disability-free life expectancy.
[d] Active life expectancy.
Source: Jitapunkul et al. (1999).

TABLE 6.5

Thailand: Ratios (per 100) of Health Expectancy to Life Expectancy By Age and Sex

	Male			Female		
	LDFLE/LE	TDFLE/LE	ALE/LE	LDFLE/LE	TDFLE/LE	ALE/LE
60–64	80.8	76.1	91.9	76.1	69.7	89.2
65–69	78.9	74.5	90.5	73.1	67.1	87.1
70–74	77.1	72.6	89.1	70.1	64.6	84.9
75–79	75.5	70.6	87.4	67.4	62.2	82.4
80+	72.4	66.7	82.2	64.0	60.3	79.1

Source: Jitapunkul et al. (1999).

remains vulnerable to recurrent crises. This has to an extent shifted the attention of the Thai Government and the public away from the issues of population ageing, and economic difficulties constrain the allocation of funds. Rapid demographic change, combined with an already alarming rate of poverty and shrinking resources in Thailand, underscores the pressing need for innovative policies that take into account the need to increase participation and social integration of older people. Poverty continues to be the greatest threat to social and economic security, affecting the ability of older people and their families to go beyond addressing basic needs. Therefore, prominent attention is mandatory to address the macroeconomic implications of population ageing in areas such as labour and capital markets, government pensions, services and traditional support systems.

Development of the First National Long-term Plan of Action for the Elderly (1986–2001)

The first provision for older persons in Thailand was the Government Welfare Institution for the Elderly, which was established in 1953. However, there were no formal national policies on ageing until 1986. The First World Assembly on Ageing held in Vienna in 1982 proposed several plans of action. The Thai Government responded by setting up the National Committee for the Elderly with the Ministry of the Interior serving as its chairperson. In 1986, the National Committee for the Elderly developed the National Long-term Plan of Action for the Elderly (1986–2001) (Knodel et al. 2000). The plan supported the implementation of government policies on care for older people and was used as a framework and guideline for activities initiated by authorized organizations such as the National Committee on Ageing of Thailand, 1986. However, data were very limited on older people in Thailand at the time the plan was being developed. Therefore, the main features of this plan were based on recommendations of the International Plan of Action on Ageing, a report by the First World Assembly on Ageing (United Nations 1983). Public and NGO participation in the plan's development was also limited.

The First National Long-term Plan of Action for the Elderly mainly targeted older persons. Its objectives were:

1. To provide older people with general knowledge on the changes of age and necessary environmental adjustments, including health care,
2. To provide older persons with the protection and support of families and communities, including other welfare services as deemed necessary
3. To support the role of older people in participation in family and other activities

4. To emphasize the responsibility of the society for older people.

Measures in the plan were confined to four aspects of life in old age, including health, education, income and employment, and social and cultural aspects. The major measures were:

1. To disseminate knowledge to older persons on self-adjustment, self-health care, prevention of disease, nutrition and proper exercise
2. To extend social welfare services for older persons, particularly for those without income or with insufficient income and with no support
3. To provide education, training or occupational counselling for the capable elderly to equip them with knowledge and skills for employment
4. To organize recreational activities for older persons to facilitate the transfer of their knowledge and experience to younger generations
5. To campaign for recognition of the importance of the extended family system and the social values of respecting and paying gratitude to ancestors and older persons
6. To cooperate with religious institutions in disseminating morals for the spiritual help of older persons, including the development of moral teaching using diverse and appropriate methods
7. To promote and support the role of communities and the private sector in providing welfare services for older persons and providing the opportunity for them to participate in various activities
8. To train personnel in caring and providing services for older persons
9. To collect basic data and to encourage study, research, monitoring and evaluation of the issues concerning older persons.

This First National Long-term Plan was announced and disseminated to government and non-governmental organizations and private corporations concerned with older persons. However, there was little progress in the state activities related to elderly organizations between 1986–1991. Research and personnel training were the outstanding achievements of the plan for the elderly during this period. In 1991, the United Nations General Assembly (resolution 46/91) adopted the United Nations Principles for Older Persons. Governments, including that of Thailand, were encouraged to incorporate these principles into their national programmes whenever possible.

Later in 1992, the Government of Thailand developed *The Essence of the Long-term Policies and Measures for the Elderly (1992–2011)* (Working Group on Policies and Main Strategies for the Support of Elderly 1992). These measures helped accelerate actions, particularly the welfare driven by state organizations. They also influenced the Eighth National Economic and Social Development Plan (1997–2001) which included a section providing social welfare benefits to older persons (Knodel et al. 2000). These welfare benefits included a living allowance to indigent elderly people, universal free health services and discounted fares for public transportation.

However, a prominent criticism of the First National Long-term Plan of Action for the Elderly (1986–2001) was that it did not have a policy on preparing people for old age (Jitapunkul and Bunnag 1997). Many feel that preparation for old age is essential in order to ensure that individuals enter old age with an acceptable quality of life. This should be a lifetime process, starting from youth and covering all critical aspects of life including health, education, income security, house and environment, and social integration.

Apart from old age preparation, suggestions for future activities related to older adults include improving self-care, boosting social participation, strengthening family values and integrating relationships, and sustaining family support for older persons. However, the role of the government in providing basic care services cannot be neglected. An important consideration in Thailand is how social security schemes, which currently cover only a fraction of the population, can take hold without duplicating the problems experienced by developed countries, particularly the problems of draining financial resources. These and other criticisms and suggestions have been seriously considered for the drafting of the Second National Long-term Plan for Older Persons (2002–2021).

Major programme developments in response to the First Long-term Plan of Action for the Elderly

Over the past ten years, since the publication of *The Essence of the Long-term Policies and Measures for the Elderly (1992–2001)* in 1992 many major programmes related to older adults have been implemented. The Department of Social Welfare (Ministry of Labour and Social Welfare) is the principal organization responsible for social service provision, including both institutional and community care. Nevertheless, formal social services mainly serve a remedial function when the family system fails to perform. At present, the Department of Social Welfare operates 20 homes for older persons and 18 centres for the elderly which provide day-care services, emergency shelter services and mobile services for older persons living in the community (Department of Social Welfare, Thailand 2001a). In 1993, the Department of Social Welfare set up a welfare fund, which provided 200 baht per month to poor, older persons. Since 1999, the monthly allowance has been increased to 300 baht per month (US$1 approximately equals 45 Thai baht). About 400,000 older persons receive this payment. In 1999, 200 "social services centres for older persons in temples" had been set up. These community centres, operated by community leaders, are able to provide only recreation activities and health promotion programmes, but not community or home care.

Many non-government organizations, such as the Thai Red Cross Society, HelpAge International, the Duangprateep Foundation, some religious organizations and several non-profit organizations, provide community care for older persons, especially those in poor and remote areas. HelpAge International has several projects which aim to support income-generating programmes in rural areas. It also funds many community services projects, including social and health services in several areas. Some non-government organizations also run institutional care programmes, including homes for older persons and nursing homes. Many private nursing homes have been set up during the decade to 2001, but most are in Bangkok. However, the exact number of these nursing homes is not known, since some nursing homes do not register with the authorities and many acute-care private hospitals have turned their wards into long-stay care facilities.

In 1994, there were 3,487 registered senior citizens' clubs in Thailand (Siripanich et al. 1996). Nevertheless, the actual number may be higher, since many clubs are not officially registered. Most senior citizens' clubs are located in state hospitals. The Senior Citizen Council of Thailand, established in 1988, supervises all registered senior citizens' clubs. The government supports the activities of these clubs through the Ministry of Public Health and the Ministry of Labour and Social Welfare.

In 1992, the Ministry of Public Health started a free health care programme for Thai older persons. Since then, older persons have been entitled to receive medical services free of charge in all state hospitals and health centres under the supervision of the Ministry of Public Health and the Bangkok Metropolitan Administration. Although there is no special in-patient service, all state-run hospitals, which have 60 beds or more, have set up geriatric clinics. These clinics are concerned with health promotion, disease prevention and acute general medical problems. They give little support for rehabilitation and do not offer home visits or social services. At present, there is no long-stay care service for older persons provided by state health care providers.

The government has promoted seniority and family values by creating an "elderly day" and a "family's day" during the Songkran festival, the traditional Thai New Year. Television and radio programmes and community ceremonies also help to promote this event nationally. Various other benefits have emerged. Public transportation support for older persons is only available for trains operated by the Royal Thai Railway Authority, a state enterprise. Older persons can receive a 50 per cent fare reduction from June to September. Education and training for health personnel, caregivers and older persons is available across the country. The government is giving full support to these activities, deemed essential for providing future services for older persons. Education and training for both health and social professionals have been set up by several organizations, including various faculties of universities, medical schools, nursing schools, the Institute of Geriatric Medicine, and the Thai Society of Gerontology and Geriatric Medicine. Nurses, physicians and social workers are the main targets. Nevertheless, there remains a severe shortage of rehabilitation personnel working with older adults.

Training programmes for family members and caregivers are provided by many organizations, including medical schools, nursing schools, universities, the Department of Social Welfare, some state-run hospitals, the Thai Red Cross Society and some non-government organizations. Non-formal educational programmes for older persons provided by the Department of Non-formal Education and the Ministry of Education give Thai older persons a chance to be educated and continue to be physically, intellectually and mentally active. Many educational courses or sessions for older persons are arranged regularly throughout the year by various organizations including government organizations, non-government organizations, private organizations and senior citizens' clubs. Many government and private organizations also provide pre-retirement programmes for their employees.

A "Declaration on Thailand's Older Persons" was announced during the United Nation's International Year of Older Persons in 1999. Non-governmental and governmental organizations participated in the preparation of this declaration. The declaration covers issues of dignity, worthiness and the protection of older persons. It was also stressed that older persons should be viewed as consistently active members of society.

The constitution of the Thai Kingdom
Since 1997, Thailand has had a new constitution which, for the first time, mentions older adults. Article 54 and Article 80 of the constitution clearly state that the government must provide assistance and welfare to older persons aged 60 and over, particularly those who lack a subsistence income or who are underprivileged. Although the emphasis here is on state actions

for the poor or underprivileged older persons, this is a crucial step in raising public awareness.

Development of the Second National Long-Term Plan for Older Persons (2002–21)

Prior to the mid-1990s, the development of national policies on ageing for Thailand had been mainly influenced and driven by United Nations recommendations. Since 1996, however, academics and institutes, with support from funding agencies, have reviewed and conducted an increasing amount of policy research towards this end. This not only provides data on the factual situation of older persons and its impact in the near future, but also provides essential data for developing a new national long-term plan for older persons (Working Group on Drafting of the Second National Long-term Plan for Older Persons 2001). During this period, key individuals, such as Dr Bunloo Siripanich, and some governmental and non-governmental organizations such as the Institute of Geriatric Medicine of the Ministry of Public Health, the Department of Social Welfare (Ministry of Labour and Social Welfare), the Society of Council of Older Persons of Thailand, and the Thai Society of Gerontology and Geriatric Medicine, have motivated the Thai Government to establish a national committee, the National Commission of the Elderly, chaired by the deputy prime minister. The committee comprises heads or representatives from various government and non-government organizations, the private sector and academic personnel. Its secretariat comprises three state organizations, the Office of the Prime Minister, the Institute of Geriatric Medicine of the Ministry of Public Health, and the Department of Social Welfare. These three agencies have a key role in drawing up national policies on ageing.

A priority task of the National Commission on the Elderly is to develop a new national long-term plan for older persons. This Second National Long-term Plan for Older Persons (NPA) was drafted and conceptualized mainly on the motivation of local institutions and individuals concerned with and interested in issues of ageing. Opinions and suggestions from the public have been collected for verifying the final version of the plan. The plan was endorsed by the Cabinet in 2002.

The Second National Long-term Plan for Older Persons was drafted using important data collected during the previous five years (Working Group on Drafting of the Second National Long-Term Plan for Older Persons 2001). The plan was drafted on the following basic concepts:

1. Security in old age means security for society.
2. General responsibility for addressing the issues related to ageing should be mainly carried out by individuals, then by families, then by communities including local authorities, and then by the government. However, the public role of the government in providing basic care services cannot be denied.
3. Life-course planning is essential for preparation for old age.
4. Preparation for old-age security is primarily the responsibility of the individual. Every person must prepare him- or herself for old-age security with support from his or her family and community. The government and the public must endorse the preparation process and act as the last resource for those who fail to have security in their late life. Old-age security includes the following:
   i)   Income security
   ii) Security in health and health care
   iii) Home and environment
   iv) Security of care during periods of dependency (family, community, and public care and services)
   v)   Rights and safety
   vi) Information and knowledge.
5. Although older persons in Thai society are no longer as highly respected as they were in the past, evidence shows that many are still playing an active role in family activities. Older persons in Thailand are still considered valuable and potential assets. Therefore, they should be encouraged to be remain integrated into society. It is essential to enhance the

contributions of older persons and diminish their image as a dependent population group.

6. Older persons should live with their families and in their communities with a reasonable quality of life.

7. The rights of older persons must be protected, especially from abuse, neglect and violence.

8. Families and communities are footholds for older persons. The national plan should aim at strengthening the capability of families and communities to support older persons appropriately. The key to success is the strength of multi-generation relationships.

9. Most older persons are not handicapped or a burden on society. Even the unlucky ones only need the support of society and the government during a certain period of their lives.

10. State welfare and services have to meet the needs of older persons who cannot stay with their families or in their communities with an acceptable quality of life.

11. The government has to encourage the private sector to participate in providing services under government supervision to protect older persons as consumers.

12. Cooperation and ongoing dialogue among non-governmental and inter-governmental, private and public sectors is required for drawing up the most effective and equitable policy for older persons.

13. The Second National Long-term Plan for Older Persons is developed with a holistic approach to prepare persons for old age and security in old age.

14. The plan must have indicators for each measure. Its overall success must be monitored using population-target indicators with appropriate time limits.

The Second National Long-term Plan for Older Persons comprises five sections:

Section 1: Strategies in the preparation for old age with quality

Section 2: Strategies for encouraging and promoting older persons

Section 3: Strategies of social security for senior citizens

Section 4: Strategies of management systems at the national level and in personnel development

Section 5: Strategies of research to support policy and programme development and of monitoring and evaluating the Second National Long-term Plan for Older Persons.

Section 1: Strategies in the preparation for old age with quality. This comprises three measures covering the following issues:

1. Extension of income security for old age covering the population in general
2. Life-long education
3. Public education on the importance and the dignity of old age.

Section 2: Strategies for encouraging and promoting older persons. The six measures are:

1. Health promotion, disease prevention and self-care among older persons
2. Enhancing the cooperation and strength of organizations and networks dealing with older persons
3. Promoting income security and employment for older persons
4. Supporting the potential and value of older persons
5. Encouraging the media to broadcast programmes for older persons and encouraging older persons to have access to various forms of information
6. Providing older persons with proper accommodation and living environments.

Section 3: Strategies for social security for senior citizens. The four measures cover:

1. Income security and employment in old age
2. Health security
3. Family caregivers and protection of the rights of older persons
4. Service systems and support networks.

Section 4: Strategies in management systems at the national level and in personnel development. This includes two measures:

1. Management systems at the national level
2. Personnel and caregiver education and training.

Section 5:   Strategies for research to support policy and programme development, and monitoring and evaluating the Second National Long-term Plan for Older Persons. Three measures cover:

1. Promoting and supporting research on older persons which focuses on policy and programme development
2. Promoting and supporting research relevant to older persons (the research should focus on policy and programme development, service improvement and other knowledge which is useful for the improvement of older persons' quality of life)
3. Developing mechanisms for continuous monitoring and evaluation of the Second National Long-term Plan for Older Persons.

The Second National Long-term Plan for Older Persons has 52 well-defined population-target indicators within appropriate time limits (determined at 5, 10, 15 and 20 years) for every measure. For monitoring the plan, three overall indexes are identified, including active life expectancy (ALE), active life expectancy–life expectancy ratio (ALE/LE) and a population ageing quality index (PAQ Index) comprising 12 indicators.

According to the Second National Long-term Plan for Older Persons, not only has the "situation of older persons" been addressed, but also other issues such as "preparation for old age for every individual", "sustaining of multi-generational relationships within Thai society" and the "contribution to the society of older persons".

At present, it is clear that in Thailand steps are being taken to develop new policies that address the changing demographic balance, but ageing still remains a low priority on the government's agenda. National laws can only be effective if adequate resources are available to implement them. Moreover, national policies need to incorporate the issue of ageing and appropriate support mechanisms for older persons into the mainstream of national social and economic planning. The government should also seek the active participation of elderly people themselves and their families, their communities and of non-governmental organizations, for guidance with research, planning and policy implementation.

The Universal Health Insurance Scheme

Currently, the government is trying to work out strategies to implement the Universal Health Insurance Scheme. Under this scheme, Thai people will receive almost all medical and health services with a 30-baht co-payment. The pilot project was launched on 1 April 2001 at hospitals run by the Ministry of Public Health in six provinces. The scheme is expected to be fully implemented by 2004. An estimated budget of 100 billion baht will be required for the project to be fully operational and the costs are estimated to rise by 2 per cent annually after inflation. This implies the costs of the scheme will exceed 150 billion baht within 10 years. Meanwhile, however, as older persons have been eligible for the free health care provided by the Ministry of Public Health since 1992, this scheme may possibly add only minimal benefits for them.

Although the financial barriers to care have arguably been relieved, there are numerous other barriers to effective health care. For example, in terms of physical accessibility, most health care facilities are concentrated in urban areas, while the majority of older persons people live in rural areas. Transportation costs are another hurdle. To eliminate the accessibility barrier, it is essential to improve the health and social care delivery system, particularly community services and mobile-service units.

Interim conclusions: national policy on ageing in Thailand

The rapid speed of population ageing in Thailand is likely to be a major constraint for the country's socio-economic development due to its contracted time of preparation to deal with the demographic consequences. Although Thai society and the government understand the essence of the National Policy on Ageing and the actions required to deal with population ageing, issues of ageing still have a low priority on the government agenda. However, development of the national policy on ageing in Thailand has been remarkable during the past fifteen years. It is notable that the principal driving forces behind the development of policy have shifted from the external (such as the United Nations) to the internal (need and vision). Therefore, the success of Thailand's national policy on ageing calls for active participation and close collaboration among governmental, non-governmental and voluntary organizations, private corporations, academia and the media. Resources and legislation are required for effective implementation of national policies. Monitoring and evaluation of the Second National Long-term Plan for Older Persons is crucial for efficient, equal and sustainable development.

Long-term care provision for older persons

As noted in Chapter 1, long-term care (LTC) is a broad term and its precise meanings are understood differently from country to country. Its narrow definition encompasses only institutional care, including nursing homes and residential homes, but more broadly it covers both institutional and community care, which emphasizes rehabilitation or maintenance support but not cure. Turner (1988) defined LTC as comprehensive, coordinated health and supportive services provided in a variety of formal and informal settings to individuals with chronically impaired function to help them attain, maintain or regain health and optimal function. Individuals of all ages can be recipients of LTC, although internationally older persons are its largest users. The range of services that comprise LTC is diverse; the continuum of care extends from non-medical, personal services to highly skilled medical care. Professional nurses, allied health professionals, para-professionals and family members can all provide LTC.

The need for LTC in Thailand

The need for long-term care for older persons in Thailand arises as a result of the rapidly growing ageing population and the declining health status of older persons. It is estimated that one in five older Thais (aged 60 and over) have some degree of disabilities according to their mobility and 6.7 per cent need assistance with personal care (see Tables 6.2 and 6.3) (Jitapunkul et al. 1999). Data on diseases or health problems which contribute to disability, obtained from the national study, have been prioritized. Stroke, osteoarthritis of the knees, blindness (mainly from cataracts), accidents and kyphoscoliosis (mainly from osteoporosis and spinal fracture) are among the high priority diseases/health problems of older Thais (Jitapunkul et al. 1999).

From the national survey, 3.4 per cent of Thai older persons have dementia (Jitapunkul et al. 2001) and its prevalence increases dramatically with age (Figure 6.3). The prevalence of

FIGURE 6.3
Thailand: Age-Specific Prevalence by Sex of Dementia Among Older Persons

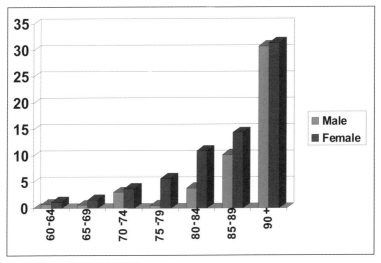

Source: Jitapunkul et al. (1999).

dementia at the age of 60–69 is only around 1 per cent, but it is more than 30 per cent at the age of 90 and over. Hence, age-specific prevalent rates of dementia among older persons in Thailand appear similar to those in more developed countries (Preston 1986; Jorm et al. 1987; Hofman et al. 1991; Ritchie and Fuhrer 1992). Around 50 per cent of the dementia among older persons is caused by Alzheimer's disease (Phanthumchinda et al. 1991). Dementia is one the most burdensome diseases for caregivers in Thailand, as elsewhere (Bunrayong 2000; Sasat et al. 2000; Rakkhanam 2000).

Table 6.6 forecasts the number of disabled and demented older persons in the next twenty years (Jitapunkul et al. 1999). In 2020, more than 700,000 older persons are likely to need some form of long-term care. Unfortunately, there is evidence of growing morbidity and disability among the Thai population, which will continue for at least fifty years unless appropriate actions are taken (Jitapunkul 2000a). This means that the number of older persons in need of special care will probably be higher than projected. Therefore, the rapid ageing of society and the increase in the proportion of those suffering from chronic illnesses and disability have exerted substantial pressure on the demand for long-term care. It is clear that the development of comprehensive LTC provision is essential for assuring an acceptable quality of life for older persons.

The principal form of LTC in Thailand is informal care provided by the family. Most older persons who need assistance with basic tasks live with their families, and families in Thailand are generally still expected to take care of their elderly members. It can be assumed that cultural values dictate that the norm is still for older persons to live with their grown-up children; there is even shame in not doing so. Although family support in the form of co-residence remains pervasive and appears not to have shown serious signs of declining over the previous two decades, given the rapid social and economic changes that Thailand has been experiencing it is uncertain whether the present level of family support will persist or whether the quality of caregiving will remain the same (Chayovan et al. 1988; Chayovan and Knodel 1996; Knodel et al. 2000).

TABLE 6.6

Thailand: Projected Numbers (and Percentage of Total Elderly Population) of Disabled Older Persons, 2010–30

	2000	2010	2020	2030
Home-bound	234,309	341,311	508,209	758,227
	(4.39%)	(4.74%)	(4.72%)	(4.79%)
Bed-bound	44,705	65,107	98,021	144,451
	(0.84%)	(0.90%)	(0.91%)	(0.91%)
Personal care dependent	350,641	499,837	741,766	1,100,754
	(6.57%)	(6.94%)	(6.89%)	(6.95%)
Suffering dementia	162,563	241,378	358,265	532,560
	(3.04%)	(3.35%)	(3.33%)	(3.36%)

Source: Jitapunkul et al. (1999).

Socio-economic changes include the decline in the number of family members, the increase in the number of working women and the migration of offsprings. Elderly women are more likely than men to lack informal care from families (Jitapunkul 1998a) and the prevalence of widowhood, divorce or separation is much higher among elderly women than among men (National Statistical Office, Thailand 1995). Three per cent of older females are single compared with 1 per cent of older men (Table 6.1). The difference is remarkable among those who are living in urban areas. The percentage of women living with their spouses is below that of men, and the differences increase with age (Table 6.7). The rate of those living alone is higher among elderly women than among elderly men (National Statistical Office, Thailand 1995) and the difference in the rates of those living alone also increases with age. Older persons living alone, particularly the very old, are usually considered a high-risk group. The main problems of living alone include having no-one to care during illness (31.6 per cent), loneliness (20.9 per cent), financial problems and the need to work (16.4 per cent) and difficulties in carrying out daily activities (17.8 per cent) (National Statistical Office, Thailand 1995). These older persons have less chance to receive informal care when they are dependent and need assistance. Moreover, a large number of older persons aged 75 and over, women in particular,

TABLE 6.7
Thailand: Residential Status of Older Persons by Age and Sex (percentages)

		Residential status			
	Alone	With Spouse and/or Others	With Children and/or Others	With Other Relatives	With Non-Relatives
Male					
60–64	2.1	55.4	41.7	0.5	1.0
65–69	2.2	47.8	47.8	0.8	1.8
70–74	2.3	47.7	46.5	0.3	3.2
75+	2.0	36.0	58.4	1.6	2.2
Total	2.2	48.7	47.0	0.7	1.9
Female					
60–64	4.4	41.9	51.7	1.1	1.5
65–69	4.0	41.3	51.9	1.3	1.6
70–74	5.1	34.8	55.2	1.7	3.4
75+	6.5	27.2	57.4	3.3	5.6
Total	4.8	37.6	53.5	1.7	2.7

Source: National Statistical Office, Thailand (1995).

live with a non-relative. These older persons may also lack appropriate caregivers.

Development of LTC policy and provision

As noted above, until recently, the meaning of long-term care has not been well understood in Thailand. As in many other places, generally, the public perceives LTC as long-term institutional care especially in nursing home and residential home, but not shelter services or home/community care services. However, the informal care provided by family has been well recognized as the main strategy of the national policy for 15 years (National Committe on Aging of Thailand, 1986). Indeed, as noted, the first National Long-term Plan mainly emphasized the informal care given by the family; however, it ignored provision needed to support the family. While the crucial role played by families in informal care has been recognized, state organizations have paid little attention to developing home/community services to assist older persons and their caregivers. Therefore, the availability of community-based services to support families providing care for older persons is very limited. Furthermore, there is no concrete plan or clear-cut measures to provide systematic care for the frail and dependent population.

The Department of Social Welfare of the Ministry of Labour and Social Welfare is mainly responsible for LTC services. Nearly all state-owned social services in Thailand are run by this organization. In terms of formal LTC provided by state organizations, social services are more advanced than health services. However, as in many countries, formal LTC services in Thailand began with institutions. The first institutional service for older persons was established in 1956 and called the Homes for Older Persons (Department of Social Welfare, Thailand 2001*a*). It provides services for low-income elderly people who were unable to stay with their families or who were without any relative to stay with. Older persons who are eligible to stay in Homes for Older Persons have to be independent in personal care and have no need of nursing care. However, when these elderly people become frailer, they may need personal or nursing care. Unfortunately, public nursing homes for older persons are not yet available in Thailand. Inevitably, older persons living in residential homes who need special care have to be taken care of by the staff of those homes. The Homes for Older Persons therefore actually provide a range of services, including shelter, residential home and nursing home functions, but do not have adequate resources for nursing care, which is their main problem.

The non-profit and for-profit private sectors have been major contributors to nursing home services during the past decade (Jitapunkul 2000b). The major contributors are private hospitals and religion-linked non-government organizations. Since there are no specific ministerial regulations for nursing homes, such homes can be registered under various categories, such as hospitals for acute treatment; and private hospitals with facilities to treat acute illnesses can convert some beds for long-stay care service immediately. Therefore, data on total numbers of nursing homes and their capacity is not available from official records. In addition, quality accreditation of nursing home services is currently crucial.

For a decade, the concept of LTC in the sense of home/ community care has been growing, and many models of community services in health and social care have been studied (Jitapunkul et al. 1996; Wongsith et al. 1996). Although the Department of Social Welfare has no concrete ideas or policy on LTC, it has been setting up social service centres for older persons since 1979. In terms of LTC, these centres provide day-care and basic rehabilitative services. Other well-established home/ community services for LTC are not available.

Nevertheless, in 2001 the Second National Long-term Plan for Older Persons will be implemented (Working Group on the Drafting of the Second National Long-term Plan for Older Persons 2001). It includes strategies on LTC provisions which cover a wide range, from promoting and supporting informal care within the family, providing health and social services for the home/ community and institutions, and developing shelter/ accommodation services and environmental adaptations to suit the activities of older persons. Moreover, under the universal coverage health care finance scheme noted earlier, primary care centres must provide community health services. This will strengthen LTC for elderly people in the future. However, over-reliance on family care and the current economic problems affecting the nation and region may suppress the progress of LTC development, particularly in home and community services and state-owned nursing homes.

Current sources of long-term care

Informal care by family

Most Thai older persons share the same house with their children (71 per cent), live in accommodation adjacent to their children's homes (9.4 per cent), or dwell in the same community with their children (7.4 per cent) (Chayovan and Knodel 1996). Among the elderly population who do not reside with their children, from 69 to 87.8 per cent are visited by their children regularly (at least once a month) (Kamnuansilpa et al. 1999; Chayovan and Knodel 1996). Indeed, tradition is strong and 93 per cent of older persons want their children to be their caregivers when they get older and need assistance (National Statistical Office, Thailand 1995). According to research survey conducted on older persons in the community, 64 per cent and 27 per cent of older persons were taken care of by their children and spouses respectively. This survey also indicated that nearly 20 per cent of caregivers were themselves also aged (National Statistical Office, Thailand 1995).

The currently available data on nursing homes and residential homes show that fewer than 4,000 older persons are presently institutionalized for LTC (Jitapunkul 2000b). Hence, almost all older persons who need LTC mainly receive informal care provided by their families and relatives. What is certain is that the proportion of those who are in need of utilizing formal care services will increase. However, the real issue regarding policy direction is how to support the informal care system in order to keep the number of elderly people needing to be placed in institutions as low as possible. The linked issue is to assure that family and relatives can provide adequate care to older people.

Home and community services
Although the main policy direction of the new National Long-term Plan for Older Persons will be to emphasize home and community-based services to enable older persons to continue living in their own homes or in the community (Working Group on Drafting of the Second National Long-term Plan for Older Persons 2001), the provision of appropriate services is very limited at present. Most available community services for older and disabled persons are not long-term provisions and are provided only on request or in emergencies.

Day-care centres. At present, there are 18 social service centres for older persons, which provide mainly day-care and rehabilitation services for LTC, run by the Department of Social Welfare (Department of Social Welfare, Thailand 2001a). Most of these centres, attached to residential homes, are able to provide services to a limited number of older persons living within a distance of 5 to 10 km. Apart from day-care and basic rehabilitation programmes, these centres also provide medical screening and treatment, counselling, recreation activities and mobile clinics.

Formal caregiver centres.   Formal caregiving centres are flourishing as businesses. They organize caregivers to look after older persons and children in a home setting. The exact number of these formal caregiver centres is not known but it estimated that there are more than 500 such centres nationally. Some institutions such as private hospitals, nursing homes, informal educational training centres and educational institutes participate in several kinds of training programmes for young women. After finishing training, some of these caregivers work in formal institutes such as hospitals and nursing homes, although a majority of these caregivers usually work as paid caregivers in the homes of older persons. The formal caregiver centres merely act as middlemen in finding families who need caregivers to look after older persons at home. There are currently no regulations or assurances of the training standards, and courses vary in length from a week to a year. This is another issue deserving public attention.

Health out-reach services.   In recent years, with the increase in awareness of the needs of older persons in community settings, post-hospital discharge services provided by public hospitals have become broader in their scope of care. New services are being provided to cater for special needs, such as the home visit programme by nurses at Ramathibodi Hospital and by nurses and volunteers at Chulalongkorn Hospital and Institute of Neurology and Hospital. However, this kind of service may be considered to operate on a very small scale and most home-visit services are only provided to elderly patients for a certain period of time, and cannot be regarded as true LTC.

During the decade to 2001, the Ministry of Public Health launched a "Home Healthcare" policy stating that a hospital should have an out-reach team, including a physician, a nurse, a social worker and a physiotherapist, to visit patients in their homes. Staff from subdistrict health centres are also supposed to visit people at home. However, the "Home Healthcare" service did not develop as anticipated. The only existing activities in some areas are community curative care for people with chronic diseases and this does not include rehabilitation or maintenance. Moreover, data from the assessment survey of the government's health services for older persons showed that fewer than one-third of older persons have ever been visited by a health care worker in their homes (Kamnuansilpa et al. 1999).

As discussed earlier in the chapter, the universal coverage scheme in health care finance is being implemented. According to the Ministry of Public Health's guidelines for its implementation, primary care units in every catchment area have to provide community and home services. Therefore, these services, particularly the "Home Healthcare" service for older persons, will be established in the near future.

Nursing homes and residential homes
Residential homes.   Residential homes for the aged are the most common and traditional service offered by governmental and non-governmental organizations. The necessity of doing so is increasingly obvious as the number of elderly who are poor and have no families increases in tandem with the total elderly population. The provision of residential care has traditionally been the domain of the Thai Government, which to meet statutory requirements should provide homes and care for homeless and destitute older persons.

The Department of Public Welfare under the Ministry of Labour and Social Welfare is a public organization mainly responsible for providing welfare services for older persons. The first residential home in Thailand, Ban Bang Khae Home for Older Persons, was established in 1956 in order to help homeless and destitute elderly people. Now, nationally, there are some 20 residential homes (Homes for Older Persons) under the supervision of the Department of Social Welfare. The distribution of the residential homes and the number of older persons living in them are shown in Table 6.8.

TABLE 6.8
Thailand: Distribution of Homes for Older Persons, and the Number (Percentage) of Residents, by Region

Region	Number of Residential Homes	Female	Male
Bangkok	2	304 (19.8)	44 (5.9)
Central	5	383 (25.0)	121 (16.3)
North	3	207 (13.5)	154 (20.7)
North East	4	259 (16.9)	138 (18.5)
East	2	210 (13.7)	118 (15.9)
South	4	170 (11.1)	169 (22.7)
Total	20	1,533 (100.0)	744 (100.0)

Source: Department of Social Welfare, Thailand (2001a).

The criteria for admission to residential homes are that elderly people have to be homeless; have no relative to live with, or be unable to live happily or peacefully with their own families; be physically healthy with no communicable diseases; and be poor or have difficulty living with their own families. The services offered in residential homes include lodging and food, clothes, other necessary consumer goods, religious activities, physical exercise and therapeutic activities for physical rehabilitation, occupational therapy, recreation activities, traditional activities, medical services, social work services, and traditional funeral services (Department of Social Welfare, Thailand 2001a). For elderly residents whose health is deteriorating (such as people with dementia and frailty), care also includes caring for daily activities (such as bathing, feeding and toileting) and basic nursing care.

There are seven residential homes, organized by non-governmental organizations, in seven provinces, Bangkok, Prathumthani, Samutprakarn, Sakolnakorn, Saraburi, Chonburi and Angthong (Department of Social Welfare, Thailand 2001b). Most residential homes are operated by non-profit or religious organizations. The main purposes are to provide food and shelter for poor, homeless and destitute elderly people.

Nursing homes.   During the past decade, there has been growing demand for rehabilitative and nursing homes for older persons convalescing or suffering from frailty or chronic illness. The state has not yet become involved in this area. These older persons are often those who have been discharged from hospitals in order to avoid overcrowding in hospitals and to mitigate the high cost of care, and who need to be taken care of in their own homes, where family members are expected to play the role of caregivers. The burden on the family for taking care of chronically ill elderly people has led to a new service that institutionalizes frail elderly people for rehabilitation and nursing care, especially in Bangkok and urban areas. As there have been no registrations or state records of nursing homes in Thailand, it is difficult to know the exact number of such homes providing care for older persons. From data currently collected by the Department of Social Welfare, there are some 10 nursing homes (providing a total of approximately 500 beds) that provide care and rehabilitation for frail elderly people whose families can afford to pay. Their expenses, without medication and special treatment, ranges from 18,000–33,900 baht per month (Department of Social Welfare, Thailand 2001b). Most nursing homes also provide short to medium-term admission for rehabilitation. Some nursing homes also provide trained caregivers for frail elderly people whose families are willing to keep them at home. Most of these rehabilitative and nursing homes are organized by the private sector and aim to serve the families of medium to high economic status.

Another trend in care provided to older persons that has emerged during the years since the 1997 economic crisis in Thailand is hospital-based care. Pressurized by the downturn of the economy after the crisis, more than 400 private hospitals were struggling for survival. Care for frail or chronically ill elderly people therefore became additional service that the private hospitals offered to the middle and high-classes, in order to increase their revenues, by turning their acute illness wards into facilities for long-stay care. These facilities may be considered as nursing homes operated by private acute-care hospitals. A flat-rate fee for hospitalization, combined with medical rounds, well-trained nursing personnel and well-equipped facilities, was attractive to families who expected a high quality of care. In

2001, there were over 50 private hospitals in Thailand providing hospital-based care for older persons (Department of Social Welfare, Thailand 2001b). In spite all of this, facilities for long-term care are effectively limited to the number of older persons and their families who can pay for the services themselves.

Innovative formal LTC programmes

In 1995, the Thai Red Cross Society developed a sheltered housing project in Thailand, and a 168-room apartment complex for independent older persons was opened in 1997. At present, 58 per cent of the available rooms are leased and only 20 per cent of the clients are living in the apartments. It seems that shelter projects like this do not meet the requirements of older persons, as independent older persons who are still active prefer to live with their offspring or spouses.

For poorer people, during the period 1992–96, a model for comprehensive health services was tested in a slum area in Bangkok, with HelpAge International funding the project. Community services for older persons included home visiting, home nursing, home rehabilitation, education and counselling and geriatric assessment at home. A small community centre was set up to provide nursing care, primary medical care, rehabilitation and a health promotion programme (Jitapunkul et al. 1996). The effectiveness of home visit and rehabilitation services were studied and have been reported (Jitapunkul 1998b; Jitapunkul et al. 1998).

In 1995, the Department of Social Welfare, with support from the United Nations Population Fund (UNFPA) developed a community service model in four selected areas. This project was aimed at strengthening the community to organize and manage community/home care for older persons (Wongsith et al. 1996). The trial was deemed a success and the model was used for implementation in setting up 200 "social service centres for older persons in temples" in 1999. However, their results were not impressive and the success rate was estimated at under 10 per cent. The reason for this failure was the inadequacy of community participation, a rigid service package which did not suit with the needs of the community and a lack of continued financial support.

In June 2001, a social service centre for older persons located in Bangkok started a trial respite service, respite care having been identified as a useful LTC support (Chapter 1). The project was to support middle-income families who were providing care for older people, and each family was requested to pay 5,000 baht a month for the service. Should the project prove to be accepted and feasible, it is planned to introduce it in other such social service centres and private residential/nursing homes.

Conclusions

The rapid growth in Thailand's ageing population, along with socio-economic changes, have led to an increase in the number of family units unable or unwilling to care for their older members. However, while the number of older persons who need formal long-term care services is increasing, neither the existing institutional care nor home/community care are adequate to support informal family care or provide acceptable care for those who cannot stay in the community, particularly among low-income families.

It is crucial that governmental policy and programmes dealing with older persons in Thailand become more focused with regard to LTC services and systems, especially when people become older, frail and increasingly dependent. Residential accommodation options, nursing homes and social security schemes for long-term care must be explicit and well-planned to cope with the projected surge in Thailand's elderly population and its increasing expectation of life. In this respect it is fortunate that the new National Long-term Plan emphasizes strengthening informal family care and the development of formal long-term care services based on the principle that older persons should live with their families. However, there are still major obstacles facing the development of LTC, such as the automatic assumption of the readiness of families to look after their older members and the current economic problems facing the country.

Bibliography

Andrews, G.R. "Research Directions in the Region: Past, Present and Future". In *Ageing in East and South East Asia,* edited by D.R. Phillips, pp. 22–35. Edward Arnold: London, 1992.

Andrews, G.R., A.J. Esterman, A.J., Braunack-Mayer, A.J. and C.M. Rungie C.M. *Aging in the Western Pacific: A Four-Country Study".* Manila: World Health Organization, Regional Office for the Western Pacific, 1986.

Antonucci, T.C. "Social Supports and Social Relationships". In *Handbook of Aging and Social Sciences* Third Edition, edited by R.H. Binstock and L.K. George, pp. 205–226. San Diego, California and London: Academic Press, 1990.

Argyle, M. "Benefits Produced by Support Social Relationships". In *The Meaning and Measurement of Social Support,* edited by H. Veiel and U. Baumann, pp. 13–32. New York: Hemisphere Publishing Corp., 1992.

Arokiasamy, J.T. "Ageing in Malaysia and Its its Problems". In *Ageing People in Transition.* Paper presented at International Symposium on a Comparative Study of Three Cases in Asia: Korea, Taiwan and Japan, Advanced Research Centre for Human Sciences, Waseda University, 1997.

_____ . "Social Problems and Care of the Elderly", *Medical Journal Malaysia* 52, no. 3 (September 1997).

Arokiasamy, J.T. and J.S.T. Teoh "Studies Concerning the Elderly in Malaysia: An Inexhaustive Compilation of Published Studies on the Care of the Elderly in Malaysia up to December 1997". The Clearing House Project, Department of Social and Preventive Medicine, University of Malaya Medical Centre, Kuala Lumpur, 1997.

Asher, M.G. "Financing Old Age in Southeast Asia: An Overview". *Southeast Asian Affairs 1996* (Singapore: Institute of Southeast Asian Studies, 1996), pp. 72–98.

_____ . "The Future of Retirement Protection in Southeast Asia". *International Social Security Review* 51, no. 1 (1998): 3–30.

Awang, H.S. "Current Programme Implementation and Evaluation". In *Proceedings of the National Seminar on Challenges of Senior Citizens Towards Vision 2020*, Kuala Lumpur, 1 October 1992.

Bae, S.S. "A Study on the Development of Dementia Management Model in Kwangmyung City, Korea". *Journal of Health Administration* 9 (1999): 30–71.

Bengston V., C. Rosenthal, and L. Burton. "Families and Ageing: Diversity and Heterogeneity". In *Handbook of Aging and the Social Sciences*, Third Edition, edited by R.H. Binstock and L.K. George, pp. 263–87. San Diego, California and London: Academic Press, 1990.

Bowling, A. *Measuring Health: A Review of Quality of Life Measurement Scales*. Buckingham: Open University Press, 1991.

Browne, C.V. *Women, Feminism and Aging*. New York: Springer, 1998.

Burgio, L., R. Allen-Burge, A. Stevens, L. Davis, and D. Marson. "Caring for Alzheimer's Disease Patients: Issues of Verbal Communication and Social Inter-action". In *The Gerontological Prism: Developing Interdisciplinary Bridges*, edited by J.F. Clair and R.M. Allman, pp. 49–74. New York: Baywood, 2000.

Butler, R.N. and H.P. Gleason. *Productive Aging*. New York: Springer, 1985.

Bunrayong W. "Family Burdens of Caring for the Demented Elderly at Home" (in Thai). *Journal of Gerontology and Geriatric Medicine* 1 (2000): 11–8.

Byun Y.C., Y.J. Han, S.H. Lee, J.H. Park, J.I. Woo, and J.H. Lee. *A Study on the Development of Dementia Management Mapping*. Seoul: Korean Institute for Health and Social Affairs, 1997.

Census and Statistics Department, Hong Kong. *Hong Kong Annual Digest of Statistics 1987–1996*. Hong Kong: Government Printer, 1996.

_____ . *Hong Kong Population Projections 1997–2016*. Hong Kong: Government Printer, 1997.

_____ . *2001 Population Census: Summary Results and Basic Tables for Constituency Areas* (5 Vols). Hong Kong: Printing Department, Hong Kong Special Administrative Region Government, 2002*a*.

_____ . *Hong Kong Population Projections 2002–2031*. Hong Kong: Printing Department, Hong Kong Special Administrative Region Government, 2002*b*.

Chan A.C.M. "An Explanatory Model for Depression Amongst the Chinese Elderly in Hong Kong — A Cognitive-Behavioural Perspective". In *Mental Health in Hong Kong 1996/97*, edited by K.Y. Mak, T. Ng, C. Chan, T.Y. Lo, and K.S. Yip, pp. 140–61. Hong Kong: Mental Health Association of Hong Kong, 1997.

Chan K.E. "Demographic and Socio-Economic Linkages in Malaysia: The Case of Demographic Ageing" In First Symposium on Gerontology 1995: *Issues and Challenges of Ageing Multidisciplinary Perspectives:* Proceedings (1995). Kuala Lumpur: Gerontology Association of Malaysia, 1996.

Chappell, N. L. *Social Support and Aging.* Toronto: Butterworths, 1992.

Chayovan N. and J.A. Knodel J. *A Report on the Survey of the Welfare of Elderly in Thailand.* Bangkok: Institute of Population Study, Chulalongkorn University, 1996.

Chayovan N., M. Wongsith M. and C. Saengtienchai. "Socio-Economic Consequences of the Aging of the Population in Thailand". IPS Publication no.161/88. Bangkok: Institute of Population Study, Chulalongkorn University, 1988.

Cheah, M. "Health Care for the Aged — Critical Issues and New Opportunities in Retirement and Nursing Homes". Paper presented at the National Conference on the Private Healthcare Industry: Shaping the Future of Malaysian Healthcare Towards the 21st Century, Petaling Jaya, March 1995.

Chen, C.Y.P., G.R. Andrews, R. Josef, K.E. Chan, and J.T. Arokiasamy. *Health and Ageing in Malaysia.* A Study Sponsored by the World Health Organization. Faculty of Medicine, University of Malaya, Kuala Lumpur, 1986.

Chen, A.J. and G. Jones. *Ageing in ASEAN — Its Socio-Economic Consequences.* Singapore: Institute of Southeast Asian Studies, 1989.

Cheung, P.L. "Population Ageing in Singapore". *Asia–Pacific Journal of Social Work 3,* no. 2 (1993): 77–89.

Chi, I. (1994) "Family Structure and Family Support of the Old Old in Hong Kong,". In *Proceedings of the International Conference on Family and Community Care, Hong Kong,* edited by Hong Kong Council of Social Service, pp. 313–18. Hong Kong:: Hong Kong Council of Social Service, 1994.

Chi, I. and J. Boey. *A Mental Health and Social Support Study of the Old Old in Hong Kong.* Hong Kong: Department of Social Work and Social Administration, University of Hong Kong, 1994.

Chi, I., P.S.F. Yip and K.K. Yu. *Elderly Suicide in Hong Kong.* Hong Kong: Befrienders International, 1997.

Chia, Y.C. "Primary Care in the Elderly". In First Symposium on Gerontology 1995: *Issues and Challenges of Ageing Multidisciplinary Perspectives:* Proceedings (1995), Gerontology Association of Malaysia, Kuala Lumpur, 1996.

Choi, J.S. *A Study on the Korean Family.* Seoul: Ilji-Sa, 1982.

Choi, S.J. "Family and Ageing in Korea: A New Concern and Challenge". *Ageing and Society* 16, no. 1 (1996): 1–25.

————— . "Approaches to Elderly Housing and Accommodation in Korea". In *Proceedings of the Asia–Pacific Regional Conference for the International Year of Older Persons, Hong Kong,* Vol. 2, pp. 238–85. Hong Kong: Hong Kong Council of Social Service, 1999*a*.

————— . "Productive Ageing in Korea". Paper presented to the International Conference of NGOs, Seoul, Korea, 10–19 October 1999, 1999*b*.

————— . "Ageing in Korea: Issues and Policies". In *Ageing in the Asia–Pacific Region: Issues, Policies, and Future Trends,* edited by D.R. Phillips, pp. 223–42. London: Routledge, 2000*a*.

————— . "Policy Tasks and Development Prospects of Current In-Home/Community Services". In *Modern In-Home/Community Care Services,* edited by the Committee for Collection of Papers to Commemorate the 70th Birthday of Mr Cho Ki-Dong. Seoul: Hongikjae, 2000*b*.

Choi, S.J. and H.K. Suh. *Aging in Korea.* Federation of the Korean Gerontological Societies. Seoul: Chung-Ang Publishers, 1995.

Chow, N. "Hong Kong: Community Care for Elderly People". In *Ageing in East and South East Asia,* edited by D.R. Phillips, pp.65–76. London: Edward Arnold, 1992.

Chung, K.H., A.J. Cho, Y.H. Oh, J.K. Byun, Y.C. Byun, and H.S. Moon. *A Research Study on the Status of the Elderly People's Life and Their Welfare Needs.* Seoul: Korea Institute for Health and Social Affairs, 1998.

Clair, J.M., W.C. Yoels, and D.A. Karp. "A Social Psychology of the Life Cycle: Interdisciplinary Policies, Perceptions and Prospects". In *The Gerontological Prism: Developing Interdisciplinary Bridges,* edited by J.M. Clair and R.M. Allman, pp. 49–74. New York: Baywood, 2000.

Clark, R.L. and J.J. Spengler. *The Economics of Individual and Population Aging.* Cambridge: Cambridge University Press, 1980.

Clegg, J. *Dictionary of Social Services.* London: Bedford Square Press, 1971.

Deloitte and Touche Consulting Group. *A Study of the Needs of Elderly People in Hong Kong for Residential Care and Community Support Services.* Hong Kong: Hong Kong Government, 1997.

Department of Social Welfare, Malaysia. *Annual Statistical Bulletin, 1995; 1996; 1997; 1998; 1999.* Kuala Lumpur: External Services Division, National Printing Department, 1995–1999.

Department of Statistics, Malaysia. *Senior Citizens and Population Ageing in Malaysia.* Population Census Monograph Series no. 4. Kuala Lumpur: National Printing Department, 1998.

_____ . *Population Distribution and Basic Demographic Characteristics*. Kuala Lumpur: Department of Statistics, 2001.

Department of Statistics, Singapore. *General Household Survey 1995: Socio-Demographic and Economic Characteristics*. Singapore: Department of Statistics, 1995.

_____ . *Key Indicators on the Population of Households, Singapore, 19/2/2001*. Website of Singapore Department of Statistics, <www.singstat.gov.sg>, 2001.

Department of Social Welfare, Thailand. *A Social Welfare for the Aged*. Bangkok: Department of Social Welfare, Ministry of Labour and Social Welfare, 2001*a*.

_____ . *A Survey of Private Organizations Providing Care and Services for the Aged*. Bangkok: Department of Social Welfare, Ministry of Labour and Social Welfare, 2001*b*.

Domingo, L.J. "Ageing and Women in Developing Countries: Examination of Issues from a Cohort Perspective". In *Population Growth and Demographic Structure: Proceedings of the U.N. Expert Group Meeting on Population Growth and Demographic Structure*. New York: United Nations, 1992.

ESCAP (Economic and Social Commission for Asia and the Pacific). *Studies on Consequence of Population Change: Malaysia*. Asian Population Studies Series no. 118. New York: United Nations, 1993.

_____ . *Population Ageing and Development: Report of the Regional Seminar on Population Ageing and Development*. Asian Population Studies Series no. 140. New York: United Nations, 1996*a*.

_____ . *Population Ageing in Asia and the Pacific*. New York: United Nations, 1996*b*.

_____ . *Approaches to Comprehensive National Policies on Ageing: Government–NGO Cooperation*. New York: United Nations, 1997.

_____ . *Macau Plan of Action on Ageing for Asia and the Pacific*. New York: United Nations, 1999.

_____ . *Ageing in Asia and the Pacific: Critical Issues in National Policies and Programmes*. SD/RW/MPAA/INF.4. Bangkok: Economic and Social Commission for Asia and the Pacific, 2001*a*.

_____ . *Review of Progress in the Implementation of the Macao Plan of Action on Ageing for Asia and the Pacific 2001*. SD/RW/MPAA/INF.5. Bangkok: Economic and Social Commission for Asia and the Pacific, 2001*b*.

_____ . *ESCAP Population Data Sheet 2001*. Bangkok: Economic and Social Commission for Asia and the Pacific, 2001*c*.

_____ . *Social Services for Older Persons: Trends and Issues in Asia and the Pacific.* SD/RW/MPAA/INF.3. Bangkok: Economic and Social Commission for Asia and the Pacific, 2001*d*.

The Edge. "Golden Oldies" in "Survey and Guide". Kuala Lumpur, 19 February 2001*a*.

_____ . "Selling to the Silver-haired" in "Survey and Guide". Kuala Lumpur, 19 February 2001*b*.

Elder, G.H., J.R. Rudkin, and M.J. Shanhan. "Psychosocial Stress over the Life Course". In *Psychosocial Stress: Perspective on Structure, Theory, Life Course, and Method,* edited by H. Kaplan, pp. 247–292. San Diego: Academic Press, 1996.

Elderly Commission, Hong Kong. *Report of the Elderly Commission 1997– 1999.* Hong Kong: Government of the Hong Kong Special Administrative Region, 2000.

_____ . *Report on Healthy Ageing.* Ad hoc Committee on Healthy Ageing, Elderly Commission, Hong Kong. Hong Kong: Printing Department, Hong Kong Special Administrative Region Government, 2001.

Employees' Provident Fund. *Employees' Provident Fund Annual Report 1999.* EPF, Malaysia, 1999.

_____ . Website: <www.kwsp.gov.my>

Encel, S. and P. Nelson. *Volunteering and Older People.* Report by the Consultative Committee on Ageing, Sydney, 1996.

Evashwick, C.J. *The Continuum of Long-term Care: An Integrated System Approach.* Albany: Delma Publishers, 1996.

Fox, L. and E. Palmer. "New Approaches to Multipillar Pension Systems: What in the World is Going On?" In *New Ideas about Old Age Security: Toward Sustainable Pension Systems in the 21st Century,* edited by R. Holzmann and J.E. Stiglitz et al., pp. 90–132. Washington, D.C.: The World Bank, 2001.

Garner, J.D. "Long-term Care". In *Encyclopedia of Social Work,* 19th Edition edited by R. Edwards et al., pp. 1625–34. Washington, D.C.: National Association of Social Workers, 1995.

Gilbert, N. and P. Terrell. *Dimensions of Social Welfare Policy,* Fourth edition. Boston: Allyn and Bacon, 1998.

Gorman, M. "Development and the Rights of Older Persons". In *The Ageing and Development Report: Poverty, Independence and the World's Older People,* edited by J. Randel, T. German and D. Ewing, pp. 3–22. London: Earthscan, 1999.

Government of Malaysia. *Seventh Malaysia Plan 1996–2000.* Kuala Lumpur: National Printing Department, 1996.

————— . *National Health and Morbidity Survey II 1996*. Kuala Lumpur: Ministry of Health, National Printing Department, 1997.

————— . *Labour Force Survey Report*. Kuala Lumpur: Department of Statistics, National Printing Department, 1998–1999.

————— . *National Senior Citizens Policy Action Plan 1999*, Kuala Lumpur: Department of Social Welfare, Ministry of National Unity and Social Development, National Printing Department, 1999.

Government of Singapore. *Singapore Census of Population*. Advanced Data Release no. 6, 2000*a*.

————— . *Singapore Census of Population*. Advanced Data Release no. 9, 2000*b*.

Harrison, J.D. "The Physical Environment: Blessing or Curse for Senior Citizens?". In *Into the Millennium of the Older Adult: Releasing Potentials and Erasing Prejudices,* Proceedings of the Regional Conference of the Gerontological Society of Singapore, 12–14 January 2001, edited by L. Wee, K. Mehta, C.Y. Leng and P.K. Tee, pp. 79–91. Singapore: The Gerontological Society of Singapore, 2001.

Hartz, G.W. and Splain, M.D. *Psychosocial Intervention in Long- term Care: An Advanced Guide for Social Workers and Nurses.* New York: Haworth Press, 1997.

Hashimoto, A. "Ageing in Japan". In *Ageing in East and South-East Asia,* edited by D.R. Phillips, pp. 36–44. London: Edward Arnold, 1992.

Health and Welfare Bureau Hong Kong. *Consultancy Study on the Review of Day Care Centres, Muiti-service Centres and Social Centres and Development of Integrated Care Services for Elders.* Study commissioned by the Health and Welfare Bureau, led by Law S.K. Hong Kong: Government of the Hong Kong Special Administrative Region, 2001.

HelpAge International. *State of the World's Older People 2002.* London: HelpAge International, 2002.

Hennessy, P. *Caring for the Frail Elderly: Policies in Evolution.* Social Policy Studies no. 19. Paris: Organization for Economic Co-operation and Development, 1996.

Heumann, L.F. and D.P. Boldy, eds. *Aging in Place with Dignity: International Solutions Relating to the Low-income and Frail Elderly.* Westport, Conn.: Praeger, 1993.

Heumann, L.F., M.E. McCall and D.P. Boldy, eds. *Empowering Frail Elderly People: Opportunities and Impediments in Housing, Health, and Support Service Delivery.* Westport, Conn.; Praeger, 2001.

Ho, K.C. and B.H Chua. *Cultural, Social and Leisure Activities in Singapore.* Census of Population Monograph no. 3. Singapore: Ministry of Community Development, 1990.

Hofman, A., W.A. Rocca, C. Brayne, et al. "The Prevalence of Dementia in Europe: a Collaborative Study of the 1980–1990 Findings". *International Journal of Epidemiology* 20 (1991): 736–48.

Hong Kong Association of Gerontology. *Position Paper of the Hong Kong Association of Gerontology.* Hong Kong: Hong Kong Association of Gerontology, 1996.

Hong Kong Council of Social Services. *Research on Expenditure Patterns of Low Expenditure Households in Hong Kong.* OXFAM and HKCSS. Hong Kong: Hong Kong Council of Social Services, 1996.

————. *Dementia Care in Hong Kong.* Task Force on Dementia Care, Elderly Division, HKCSS. Hong Kong: Hong Kong Council of Social Services, 1998.

Hong Kong Hospital Authority. *Hospital Authority Statistical Report 1998–99.* Hong Kong: Hospital Authority, 2000.

Howe, A. "Changing the Balance of Care: Australia and New Zealand" . In *Caring for Frail Elderly People: Policies in Evolution,* edited by P. Hennessy. Social Policy Studies no. 19. Paris: Organization for Economic Co-operation and Development, 1996.

Howe, A. and D.R. Phillips, *National Policies on Ageing: Why Have Them?* Invited Symposium, World Congress of Gerontology, International Association of Gerontology, Vancouver, July 2001.

Hutten, J.B.F. and A. Kerkstra, eds. *Home Care in Europe: A Country-specific Guide to its Organization and Financing.* Aldershot: Arena, 1996.

Hyun, O.S. "A Comparative Study on the Formulation Process of Social Welfare Policy for the Aged in Korea and Japan". Ph.D. dissertation, Department of Social Welfare, Seoul National University, 1992.

International Federation of Ageing. IFA Montreal Declaration: 4th Global Conference, <www.ifa-fiv.org/menu1.htm>, 1999.

International Labour Organization. *Early and Partial Retirement in Europe and the United States.* Briefing noted for the Senate Special Committee on Ageing, Washington D.C., 25 July 1997.

Inter-Ministerial Committee on the Ageing Population, Singapore. *Report of the Inter-Ministerial Committee on the Ageing Population.* Singapore: Ministry of Community Development, 1999.

Inter-Ministerial Committee on Health Care for the Elderly, Singapore. *Report of the Inter-Ministerial Committee on Health Care for the Elderly.* Singapore: Ministry of Health, 1999.

Jalal, H. "Future Strategies in Health Care for the Elderly in Malaysia". In *First Symposium on Gerontology 1995: Issues and Challenges of Ageing Multidisciplinary Perspectives:* Proceedings. Gerontology Association of Malaysia, Kuala Lumpur, 1996.

Jitapunkul, S. *Elderly Women : A Current Status.* Bangkok: Thai Society of Gerontology and Geriatric Medicine, 1998*a*.

——— . "A Randomised Controlled Trial of Regular Surveillance in Thai Elderly Using a Simple Questionnaire Administered by Non-Professional Personnel", *Journal of Medical Association of Thailand* 81 (1998*b*): 352–56.

——— . "Expansion of Morbidity: a Hypothesis Originated from a Study among Thai Elderly", (in Thai) *Journal Gerontology and Geriatric Medicine* 1 (2000*a*): 42–49.

——— . *Current Status of Thai Older Persons and National Actions on Ageing* (in Thai). Bangkok: Faculty of Medicine, Chulalongkorn University, 2000*b*.

Jitapunkul, S., and S. Bunnag. *Ageing in Thailand: 1997.* Bangkok: Thai Society of Gerontology and Geriatric Medicine, 1997.

Jitapunkul, S., S. Bunnag, S. and S. Ebrahim. *Care for the Elderly in Klong Toey Slum.* CES project: final report for HelpAge International. Bangkok: Faculty of Medicine, Chulalongkorn University, 1996.

——— . "Effectiveness and Cost Analysis of Community-based Rehabilitation Service in Bangkok". *Journal of Medical Association of Thailand* 81 (1998): 572–78.

Jitapunkul, S., N. Chayovan, and S. Yodpetch, eds. *Elderly in Thailand: An Extensive Review of Current Data and Situation, and Policy and Research Suggestions* (in Thai), Bangkok: The Thailand Research Fund, 2001.

Jitapunkul, S., C. Kunanusont, W. Phoolcharoen, and P. Suriyawongpaisal. *Health Problems of Thai Elderly (A National Survey)* (in Thai). Bangkok: National Health Foundation and Ministry of Public Health, 1999.

——— . "Prevalence Estimation of Dementia among Thai Elderly: a National Study". *Journal of Medical Association of Thailand* 84 (2001): 461–67.

Jitapunkul, S., S. Yodpetch, M. Pananiramai, et al. *A Future Study of Elderly Population, Welfare and Service System in the Next 10 Years* (in Thai). Bangkok: Department of Medicine, Faculty of Medicine, Chulalongkorn University, 2000.

Joaquin-Yasay, C. "Creating Awareness of the Issues and Problems of the Elderly Among Planners and Policy Makers". In *Implications of Asia's Population Future for Older People in the Family.* Report and selected background papers from the Expert Group Meeting on The Implications of Asia's Population Future for Family and the Elderly, 25–28 November 1996. New York: United Nations, 1996.

Johnson, P. and J. Falkingham. *Ageing and Economic Welfare*. London: Sage Publications, 1992.

Jorm, A.F., A.E. Korten, and A.S. Henderson, "The Prevalence of Dementia: a Quantitative Integration of the Literature". *Acta Psychiatratrica Scandinavica* 76 (1987): 456–79.

Kagawa-Singer, M. "Diverse Cultural Beliefs and Practice about Death and Dying in the Elderly". In *Cultural Diversity and Geriatric Care: Challenges to the Health Professions*, edited by D. Wieland, D. Benton, B.J.D. Kramer, and G.D. Dawson, pp. 101–115. New York: Haworth, 1994.

Kahana, E. "Long-term Care Facilities". In *Encyclopedia of Sociology*, Second edition, edited by E.F. Borgatta and R.J.V. Montgomery, pp. 1663–83. New York: Macmillan Reference, 2000.

Kamnuansilpa, P., S. Wongthanavasu, J. Bryant, and A. Promno. *Health Policy Evaluation for the Elderly Population* (in Thai). Khon Kaen: University of Khon Kaen, 1999.

_____ . "An Assessment of the Thai Government's Health Services for the Aged". *Asia–Pacific Population Journal* 15, no. 1 (2000)): 3–18.

Kane R.L. and R.A. Kane, eds. *Assessing Older Persons: Measures, Meaning and Practical Applications*. New York: Oxford University Press, 2000.

Karim, H.A. "The Elderly in Malaysia: Demographic Trends". *Medical Journal of Malaysia* 52, no. 3 (September 1997): 206–12.

Kart, G.S. *The Realities of Aging: An Introduction to Gerontology*, Fifth edition. Allyn and Bacon: Needham Heights, 1997.

Kim, I.K. "Demographic Transition and Population Aging in Korea". *Korea Journal of Population and Development* 25, no. 1 (1996): 27–40.

King, S. "Role and Functions of Non-Governmental Organizations: Provision of Community-Based Services for the Elderly; Enhancing National Capacity". In *Implications of Asia's Population Future for Older People in the Family*. Report and selected background papers from the Expert Group Meeting on the Implications of Asia's Population Future for Family and the Elderly, 25–28 November 1996. New York: United Nations Publications, 1996.

Kinsella, K. "Demographic Dimensions of Ageing in East and Southeast Asia". In *Ageing in the Asia–Pacific Region: Issues, Policies, and Future Trends*, edited by D.R. Phillips, pp. 35–50. London: Routledge, 2000.

Kinsella, K. and V.A. Velkoff. *An Aging World: 2001*. US Census Bureau, Series P95/011. Washington, D.C.: US Government Printing Office, 2001.

Kleunen, A.V. and Wilner, M. "Who will Care for Mother Tomorrow?" *Journal of Aging and Social Policy* 11, no. 2/3 (2001): 115–26.

Knodel, J., N. Chayovan, S. Graisurapong, and C. Suraratdecha. "Ageing in Thailand: An Overview of Formal and Informal Support". In *Ageing in the Asia–Pacific Region: Issues, Policies and Future Trends*, edited by D.R. Phillips, pp. 243–66. London: Routledge, 2000.

Knodel, J. and N. Debavalya. "Living Arrangements and Support among the Elderly in Southeast Asia". *Asia Pacific Population Journal* 12, no. 4 (1997): 5–17.

Knodel, J., M. VanLandingham, C. Saengtienchai, and W. Im-em. "Older People and AIDS: Quantitative Evidence of the Impact in Thailand". *Social Science and Medicine* 52, no. 9 (2001): 1313–27.

Kumar, R.V. "The Role of Employees Provident Fund (EPF) in Financing Old Age in Malaysia". In *Proceedings of the 1996 Celebrations: National Day for the Elderly*, 17–27 October 1996. Kuala Lumpur, 1997.

————— . "Old Age Financial Security for the Self-Employed". Paper presented at the seminar on Financial Security in Old Age, 9–10 October 1999, Petaling Jaya.

Kvale, J. N. "Health Care as an Expression of Culture". In *First Symposium on Gerontology 1995: Issues and Challenges of Ageing Multidisciplinary Perspectives: Proceedings (1995)*. Gerontology Association of Malaysia, Kuala Lumpur, 1996.

Kwon, J.D. *Actual Conditions of Support for the Elderly with Dementia and Strategic Measures to the Conditions*. Seoul: Korea Institute for Health and Social Affairs, 1994.

Langlais, K.J. *Managing with Integrity for Long term Care: The Key to Success for Building Stability in Staffing*. New York: McGraw-Hill, 1997.

Lee, W.K.M. "Economic and Social Implications of Aging in Singapore". *Journal of Aging and Social Policy* 10, no. 4 (1999): 73–92.

————— . "The Feminization-of-Poverty in an Aged Population in Singapore". In *Ageing, Gender and Family in Singapore, Hong Kong and China*, edited by K.W.K. Law, pp. 75–91. Taiwan: Program for Southeast Asian Studies, Academica Sinica, 2001*a*.

————— . "New Patterns of Poverty in Hong Kong: An Assessment of Current Social Security Provisions". In *Ageing, Gender and Family in Singapore, Hong Kong and China*, edited by K.W.K. Law, pp. 93–116. Taiwan: Program for Southeast Asian Studies, Academica Sinica, 2002*b*.

Leung, E.M.F. "Long-term Care Issues in the Asia–Pacific region". In *Ageing in the Asia–Pacific Region: Issues, Policies and Future Trends*, edited by D.R. Phillips, pp. 82–92. London: Routledge, 2000.

Leung, E.M.F. and M. Lo. " Social and Health Status of Elderly People in Hong Kong". In *The Health of the Elderly in Hong Kong*, edited by S.K. Lam, pp. 43–61. Hong Kong: University of Hong Kong Press, 1997.

Liu, E. and E. Wong. *Health Care for Elderly People.* Research and Library Services Division, Hong Kong Provisional Legislative Council Secretariat. Hong Kong: Provisional Legislative Council Secretariat, 1997.

Liu, W. and H. Kendig. *Who Should Care for the Elderly? An East–West Value Divide*. Singapore: Singapore University Press and World Scientific Publications, 2000.

Liu, W., and R.P.L. Lee, E.S.H. Yu, J.J. Lee and S.G. Sun. *Health Status, Cognitive Functioning and Dementia among Elderly Community Population in Hong Kong*. Faculty of Social Sciences, Hong Kong Baptist College, 1993.

LTC Policy Planning Committee, Ministry of Health and Welfare, Korea. *A Study on Comprehensive Planning for Long-term Care*. Kwachun, Ministry of Health and Welfare, 2000.

Low, L. and T.L. Ngiam. "The Underclass among the Overclass". In *Singapore: Towards a Developed Status,* edited by L. Low. Singapore: Oxford University Press, 1999.

MPKSM (Majlis Pusat Kebajikan Semenanjung Malaysia). Various Records, and *Program Report* 2000.

Mehta, K. "Social Security and Economic Well-being of Older Persons in ASEAN: The Singapore Scenario". In *Proceedings of the 1996 Celebrations: National Day for the Elderly,* 17–27 October 1996. Kuala Lumpur, 1997*a*.

———— . "The Development of Services for the Elderly in Singapore: An Asian Model". *Asia–Pacific Journal of Social Work 7*, no. 2 (1997*b*): 32–45.

———— ."Promoting Multigenerational Relationships in Asia and the Pacific". In *Promoting a Society for All Ages in Asia and the Pacific,* edited by the Economic and Social Commission for Asia and the Pacific (ESCAP), pp.56–80. New York: United Nations, 1999.

———— . "Caring for the Elderly in Singapore". In *Who Should Care for the Elderly? An East–West Value Divide*, edited by W.T. Liu and H. Kendig, pp. 249–68. Singapore: National University of Singapore Press and World Scientific Publishing, 2000.

Mehta, K. and M.B. Blake. "The Ageing Experience of Singaporean Women". In *Untapped Resources: Women in Ageing Societies Across Asia,* edited by K. Mehta, pp. 41–58. Singapore: Times Academic Press, 1997.

Mehta, K. and V. Joshi. "The Long Journey: Stress among Family Carers of Older Persons in Singapore." Paper presented at the Conference on Families in the Global Age: New Challenges Facing Japan and Singapore, Singapore, 4–6 October 2000.

Mehta K. and S. Vasoo. "Community Programmes and Services for Long-Term care for the Elderly in Singapore: Challenges for Policy-makers". *Asian Journal of Political Science* 8, no. 1 (2000): 125–40.

Mende, S. *Ageing in My Own Place: Home Care for Older People in the Asia–Pacific Region.* London: HelpAge International, 2001.

Ministry of Finance, Malaysia. *Economic Report (Annual).* Kuala Lumpur: National Printing Department, 1995–2000.

Ministry of Health, Singapore. *Towards Better Heath Care: Main Report of the Review Committee on National Health Policies.* Singapore: Ministry of Health, 1992.

Ministry of Health et al., Singapore. *The National Survey of Senior Citizens in Singapore 1995.* Singapore: Ministry of Health, Ministry of Community Development, Department of Statistics, Ministry of Labour and National Council of Social Service, 1996.

Ministry of Health and Welfare, Korea. *Health and Welfare Vision 2010* (in Korean). Kwachun: Ministry of Health and Welfare, 2000a.

_____ . *A Report on National Health and Nutrition Survey* (in Korean). Kwachun: Ministry of Health and Welfare, 2000b.

_____ . *White Paper of Health and Welfare* (in Korean). Kwachun: Ministry of Health and Welfare, 2000c.

_____ . *White Paper of Health and Welfare* (in Korean). Kwachun: Ministry of Health and Welfare, 2001a.

_____ . *Guideline of National Government's Financial Support for the Elderly Health and Welfare in 2001* (in Korean). Kwachun: Ministry of Health and Welfare, 2001b.

_____ . *A Report of Comprehensive Measures on Financial Stabilization of National Health Insurance and New Medicare System to Define Roles of Medical Doctors and Pharmacists* (in Korean). Report issued by the Ministry of Health and Welfare, 2001c.

Moroney, R. *The Family and State.* London: Longman, 1976.

Mui, A.C., N.G. Choi, and A. Monk. *Long-Term Care and Ethnicity.* Westport, Con: Greenwood Press, 1998.

Muller, C.F. *Health Care and Gender.* New York: Russell Sage Foundation, 1992.

Murphy, E. "Social Factors in Late Life Depression" In *Affective Disorders in the Elderly,* edited by E. Murphy, pp. 79–96. London: Churchill Livingstone, 1986.

National Committee on Ageing of Thailand. *National Long-term Plan for the Elderly in Thailand, 1986–2001.* Bangkok: National Committee on Ageing of Thailand, 1986.

National Statistical Office, Korea. *Population Estimates (1960–2030).* Website: <www.nso.go.kr>, 2001.

National Statistical Office, Thailand. *Report of the 1994 Survey of Elderly in Thailand.* Bangkok: National Statistical Office, Office of the Prime Minister; 1995.

Ng, A.C.Y., D.R. Phillips, and W.K.M. Lee. "Persistence and Challenges to Filial Piety and Informal Support of Older Persons in a Modern Chinese Society: A Case Study in Tuen Mun, Hong Kong". *Journal of Aging Studies* 16 (2002): 135–53.

Ngan R.M.H., E.M.F. Leung, A.Y.H. Kwan, W.T. Yeung, and A.M.L. Chong. *A Study of the Long Term Care Needs, Patterns and Impact of the Elderly in Hong Kong.* Department of Applied Social Studies, City University of Hong Kong, 1996.

Nor Aini. "Health Care of the Elderly in Malaysia". In *Proceedings of the 1996 Celebrations: National Day for the Elderly, 17–27* October 1996. Kuala Lumpur, 1997.

OECD (Organization for Economic Co-operation and Development). *Ageing in OECD Countries: A Critical Policy Challenge.* Paris: OECD, 1997.

Ogawa, N. "Changing Needs for Public Support to Families Caring for the Elderly". In *Ageing and the Family*, pp. 221–27. New York: United Nations, 1994.

Ogawa, N., N.O. Tsuya, M. Wongsith, and E. Choe. "Health Status of the Elderly and their Labor Force Participation in Developing Countries along the Asia–Pacific Rim". NUPRI Reprint Series no. 51, March 1994, from *Human Resources in Development along the Asia-Pacific Rim (1993)*, pp. 349 –72 , 1994.

Park, C.H. and H.J. Koh. "A Research on Ethiological Classification and Prevalence Rate of Senile Dementia in a Myun Area, Youngil-kun, Kyoungpuk Province". *Neuropsychiatry* 30 (1991): 885–91.

Park, T.R. *Welfare of the Elderly: Theories and Practice* (in Korean). Kyungsan: Taegu University Press, 1999.

Phanthumchinda, K., S. Jitapunkul, C. Sitthi-Amorn, S. Bunnag, and S. Ebrahim. "Prevalence of Dementia in an Urban Slum Population in Thailand: Validity of Screening Methods". *International Journal of Geriatric Psychiatry* 6 (1991): 639–46.

Phillips, D.R. *Epidemiological Transition in Hong Kong: Changes in Health and Disease since the Nineteenth Century.* Research Monographs no. 75, Centre of Asian Studies, University of Hong Kong, 1988*a*.

_____ . "Accommodation for Elderly Persons in Newly Industrializing Countries: the Hong Kong Experience". *International Journal of Health Services* 18, no. 2 (1988*b*): 255–79.

_____ . *Health and Health Care in the Third World*. London: Longman, 1990.

_____ , ed. *Ageing in East and South-East Asia*. London: Edward Arnold, 1992.

_____ . "Long-term Care". In *Encyclopedia of Sociology*, Second edition, edited by E.F. Borgatta and R.J.V. Montgomery, pp. 1652–63. New York: Macmillan Reference, 2000*a*.

_____ , ed. *Ageing in the Asia–Pacific Region: Issues, Policies and Future Trends*. London: Routledge, 2000*b*.

Phillips, D.R. and H.P. Bartlett. "Ageing Trends — Singapore". *Journal of Cross-Cultural Gerontology* 10, no. 4 (1995): 349–56.

Phillips, D.R. and A.G.O. Yeh, eds. *Environment and Ageing: Environmental Policy, Planning and Design for Elderly People in Hong Kong*. Hong Kong: Centre of Urban Planning and Environmental Management, University of Hong Kong, 1999.

Phua, K.H. "Financing Health and Long-term Care for Ageing Populations in the Asia–Pacific Region". In *Ageing in the Asia–Pacific Region*, edited by D.R. Phillips, pp. 93–112. London: Routledge, 2000.

Phua, K.H. and M.T. Yap. "Financing Health Care in Old Age". In *Choices in Financing Health and Old Age Security*, edited by N. Prescott. World Bank Discussion Paper No. 392, pp. 33–42. Washington, D.C.: The World Bank, 1998.

Preston, G.A.N. "Dementia in elderly Elderly Adults: Prevalence and Institutionalization". *Journal of Gerontology* 41 (1986): 261–7.

Rakkhanam, R. "Care for Older Persons with Dementia by Families: Burden and Needs" (in Thai). *Journal of Gerontology and Geriatric Medicine* 1 (2000): 31–7.

Rhee, K.O. "Long-term Care Needs of the Elderly in Seoul and Policy Implications". In *Gerontological Approaches to Care for the Aged in the 21st Century*, edited by S.J. Choi, pp. 519–27. Seoul: Organizing Committee for the 6th Asia/Oceania Regional Congress of Gerontology, 1999.

Rhee, K.O., H.B. Cha, S.J. Choi, H.S. Yoon, H.K. Suh, and K.S. Park. *Needs of the Elderly Under Long-term Care and Their Family's Care Burden* (in Korean). Research Report supported by Yoohan Kimberly Ltd., Korea, 1999.

Ritchie, K. and R. Fuhrer. "A Comprehensive Study of the Performance of Screening Tests for Senile Dementia using Receiver Operating

Characteristics Analysis". *Journal of Clinical Epidemiology* 45 (1992): 627–37.

Ruzicka, L.T. "Suicide in Countries and Areas of the ESCAP Region". *Asia–Pacific Population Journal* 13, no. 4 (1998): 55–74.

Sasat, S., R.M. Bryar, and A.J. Newens. "Care of Demented Older Persons by Families in Thailand" (in Thai). *Journal of Gerontology and Geriatric Medicine* 1(2000): 15–24.

Seoul National University. *A Study on Dementia Management Business.* Study Report. Seoul: Seoul National University, 1995.

Shantakumar, G. "The Aged in Singapore". *Census of Population, 1990 Monograph* no. 1. Singapore: National Printers, 1994.

———. "Ageing in the City–State Context: Perspectives from Singapore". *Ageing International* 25, no. 1 (1999): 46–58.

Sherraden, M. "Provident Funds and Social Protection: the Case of Singapore". In *Alternatives to Social Security: A International Inquiry,* edited by J. Midgley and M. Sherraden, pp. 33–59. London: Auburn House, 1997.

Sherraden, M., S. Nair, S. Vasoo, T.L. Ngiam, and M. Sherraden. "Social Policy Based on Assets: the Impact of Singapore's Central Provident Fund". *Asian Journal of Political Science* 3, no. 2 (1995): 112–33.

Sidell, M. *Health in Old Age: Myth, Mystery and Management.* Buckingham: Open University Press, 1995.

Siripanich, B., C. Tirapat, M. Singhakachin, P. Panichacheewa, and P. Pradabmuk. *A Research Report on the Senior Citizen Clubs: A Study of the Appropriate Model.* Bangkok: Senior Citizen Council of Thailand, 1996.

Smith, P. *Evaluating the Quality of Life in Singapore: Some Explorations in Economic and Social Measurement.* Singapore: Centre for Advanced Studies, National University of Singapore, 1994.

Social Welfare Department, Hong Kong. Website on elderly service information: <www.info.gov.hk/swd/html_eng/ser_sec/ser_elder/index.html>

Straits Times, Sunday Review, 18 September 1994.

Straits Times, 7 August 2000.

Straits Times, 24 August 2000.

Straits Times, 13 January 2001.

Straits Times, 23 February 2001.

Straits Times, 21 May 2001.

Sushama, P.C. "Health and Welfare Services for Elderly People in Malaysia". In *Ageing in East and South-East Asia,* edited by D.R. Phillips, pp. 167–184. London: Edward Arnold, 1992.

Tan, P.C. "Family Changes and the Elderly in Asia" In *The Ageing of Ageing of Asian Population*s, Proceedings of the United Nations Round Table on the Ageing of Asian Populations, Bangkok, 4–6 May 1992. New York: United Nations 1994.

Tan, P.C., S.T. Ng, N.P. Tey, and A. Halimah. "Evaluating Programme Needs of Older Persons in Malaysia". Kuala Lumpur: Faculty of Economics and Administration, University of Malaya, 1999.

Tarmugi, A. "Opening Address by the Minister for Community Development and Sports". In *Into the Millennium of the Older Adult: Releasing Potentials and Erasing Prejudices*, Proceedings of the Regional Conference of the Gerontological Society of Singapore, 12–14 January 2001, edited by L. Wee, K. Mehta, C.Y. Leng and P.K. Tee, pp. 3–5. Singapore: The Gerontological Society of Singapore, 2001.

Teo, P. "The National Policy on Elderly People in Singapore". *Ageing and Society* 14 (1994): 405–27.

Tey, N.P. "Social Equity: Policies and Programmes Affecting Older People in Malaysia". Paper presented at the 22nd Federation of ASEAN Economic Associations (FAEA) Conference on Southeast Asia Beyond 2000: Human Dimension, Kuala Lumpur, 1997.

Tinker, A. *Older People in Modern Society*, Fourth Edition. London: Longman 1996.

Tout, K. *Ageing in Developing Countries.* New York: Oxford University Press, for HelpAge International, 1989.

Tung, C.H. *Policy Address 2000.* Hong Kong: Government of the Hong Kong Special Administrative Region, 2000.

Turner, T.A. "The Role of Advocacy Organization". In *Strategies for Long-term Care*, edited by P.G. Maralgo, pp. 367–82. New York: National League of Nursing, 1988.

United Nations. *International Plan of Action on Ageing.* New York: United Nations, 1983.

_____ . *The Ageing of Asian Populations.* New York: United Nations Publications, 1994.

_____ . *International Plan of Action on Ageing and United Nations Principles for Older Persons.* New York: United Nations, 1998.

_____ . *Human Development Report 1999.* New York: Oxford University Press, 1999*a*.

_____ . (Department of Economics and Social Welfare). *World Population Prospects, The 1998 Revision.* New York: United Nations 1999*b*.

_____ . *Human Development Report 1999.* New York: Oxford University Press, 1999*c*.

_____ . *Madrid International Plan of Action on Ageing 2002*. Second World Assembly on Ageing, Madrid, United Nations, 2002. Website: <www.un.org/ageing/coverage/index.html>

United States Bureau of Census. (International Data Base) Website: <www.census.gov/ipc/www/idbnew.html>

Vasoo, S., T.L. Ngiam, and P. Cheung. "Singapore's Ageing Population: Social Challenges and Responses". In *Ageing in the Asia–Pacific Region: Issues, Policies and Future Trends,* edited by D.R. Phillips, pp. 174–93. London: Routledge, 2000.

Wenger, G.C. *Understanding Support Networks and Community Care.* Aldershot: Athenaeum Press Ltd., 1994.

Whang, N., J.K. Choi, Y.S. Kim, J.J. Kim, B.M. Yang, S.N. Yoon and I.S. Chang. *Model Development and Systemization of Hospital-based Home Health Care*. Seoul: Korea Institute for Health and Welfare, 1999.

Williams, E.I. "Care of Older People in the Community" In *First Symposium on Gerontology 1995: Issues and Challenges of Ageing Multidisciplinary Perspectives*. Proceedings Kuala Lumpur: Gerontology Association of Malaysia, 1996.

Wongsith, M., S. Siriboon, and A. Entz. "Community Participation in Providing Care, Services and Activities for Thai Elderly: Preliminary Rreport". IPS publication no.244/96. (1996). Bangkok: Institute of Population Studies, Chulalongkorn University, 1996.

Working Group on Drafting of the Second National Plan Long-term for Older Persons. *The Draft of the Second National Plan for Older Persons (2002–2021)*. Bangkok: Drafting Committee of the Second National Plan for Older Persons, National Commission on the Elderly, 2001.

Working Group on Policies and Main Strategies for the Support of the Elderly. *The Essence of Long-term Policies and Measures Plan for the Elderly, 1992–2011* (in Thai). Bangkok: Office of the Prime Minister, 1992.

World Bank. *Averting the Old Age Crisis: Policies to Protect the Old and Promote Growth.* New York: Oxford University Press, 1994.

World Health Organization. *Guidelines for National Policies and Programme Development for Health of Older Persons on the Western Pacific Region.* Geneva: World Health Organization, 1998.

Yamasaki, S. "Long-Term Care Insurance: The Japanese Experience". Presented at the Ministry of Community Development and Sports, Singapore, on 4 May 1999.

Yeo C.T. "Keynote Address by the Minister for Health and for the Environment, Singapore". *Conference on Choices in Financing Health Care and Old Age Security.* World Bank Discussion Paper, no. 392 (1997): 1–3.

Yuen, C. "Implementation of the Gate-keeping Mechanism: An Experience Sharing". Paper presented at the Regional Conference, *Into the Millennium of the Older Adult: Releasing Potentials and Erasing Prejudices*, Gerontological Society of Singapore, Singapore, 12–14 January 2001.

Index